Anne Woodham is the Mind & Body Editor of
Good Housekeeping, and is a freelance writer specialising in
health, education and women's issues. She is also the author of
LQM: Beating Stress at Work (also published by the Health
Education Authority).

D07755766

HEA GUIDE TO COMPLEMENTARY MEDICINE AND THERAPIES

Anne Woodham

Published in 1994
Health Education Authority
Hamilton House
Mabledon Place
London WC1H 9TX

© Anne Woodham 1994

ISBN 1 85448 903 8

A CIP catalogue record for this book is available from the
British Library.

Anne Woodham has asserted her right under the Copyright, Designs
and Patents Act, 1988, to be identified as Author of this Work.

The views expressed in this book are those of the author and not
necessarily those of the Health Education Authority.

Typesetting by Type Generation
Printed in Great Britain by The KPC Group, London and Ashford, Kent

CONTENTS

ACKNOWLEDGEMENTS

I am deeply grateful to the people who have contributed to the making of this book, for their time in reading and checking material, for their suggestions (always an improvement), their advice (always good) and their help in researching the many pieces of information.

An enormous thank you to Dr David Peters, physician, osteopath, homeopath, chair of the British Holistic Medical Association and course director in Therapeutic Bodywork, Centre for Community Care and Primary Health, University of Westminster. Not only did he read – and comment on – the manuscript, but the ratings of the therapies are his inspired suggestion. Thanks also to Simon Fielding, chair of the General Council and Register of Osteopaths and Special Adviser to Department of Health on non-conventional medicine for his valuable comments on the manuscript.

Thanks also to Maura Bright of the Council for Acupuncture, Matthew Bennett of the British Chiropractic Association, registered Rolfer Jennie Crewdson, t'ai chi ch'uan teacher Andy Fretwell, April Furnival of the Polarity Therapy Council, nutritional therapist Linda Lazarides, massage therapist Clare Maxwell-Hudson, medical herbalists Michael and Anne McIntyre, naturopath Roger Newman-Turner, cranial osteopath Caroline Penn, David Repard of the Confederation of Healing Organisations, the Shiatsu Society and Robert Tisserand of the Aromatherapy Organisations Council.

And finally, but not least, thanks to indefatigable researchers Jemima Gibbons and Catharine Robinson, and to Linda Gray, assistant editor (family and health) at Good Housekeeping.

FOREWORD

Complementary therapy has made major advances since the first BMA report in 1986. This first report suggested that the medical profession was likely to reject many of the claims made on behalf on complementary medicine. Since then research and clinical outcome papers have appeared almost weekly in orthodox medical journals. A Chair of Complementary Medicine was established in Exeter University. An MA in Therapeutic Bodywork is currently organised at the University of Westminster and there are plans for further postgraduate courses. The Osteopathy Bill was enacted through Parliament in 1993 and several health authorities have made available complementary therapy service for patients through the NHS. Fundholders have purchased the services of massage therapists, osteopaths, homeopaths and practitioners of traditional Chinese Medicine. The Labour Party have recently released their own plans for complementary therapy *(Facilitation not Prescription)* and have suggested that ring-fenced money will be made available for future research and training in Complementary Therapy.

All this progress could not have been predicted when HRH the Prince of Wales made his valedictory remarks as the President of the BMA in 1983. He said:

> Human nature is such that we are frequently prevented from seeing that what is taken for today's unorthodox is probably tomorrow's convention.

It would appear that complementary medicine is almost becoming today's orthodoxy, so a few cautious words are required.

It is important for the public to appreciate that very few, if any, of the serious chronic disorders to which we are prone - arthritis, asthma, diabetes, cancer – have been 'cured' by complementary medicine. That patients derive much benefit from many of these therapies there is no doubt, but I know of only one study that indicates that complementary therapy has any effect on the life-span of a patient with breast cancer: that study has yet to be repeated successfully. Complementary therapists must therefore be careful not to raise false hopes for that surely will undo much of the progress that has been made.

The author of this book is to be congratulated for providing an easy and accessible body of information for patients and professionals alike, and I look forward to its being circulated to all General Practitioners.

Professor Patrick Pietroni FRCGP MRCP DCH

INTRODUCTION

'My wife sent me to a healer when my injured knee wouldn't get better. He held his hands a few inches away from my leg, and I felt a kind of warmth. I've been able to walk on it ever since.'

'We tried everything for my daughter's eczema, but nothing seemed to work. Finally we took her along to a Chinese herbal doctor that friends recommended. She gave her this revolting concoction to drink, but it seemed to do the trick. Her skin has practically cleared up.'

It is stories like these that are encouraging thousands of Britons to turn – or at least to think of turning – to complementary medicine and alternative therapies. Three-quarters of the British public, according to a recent survey, would like to see treatments such as homeopathy and osteopathy available on the NHS, despite the fact that only three out of ten people have actually tried complementary medicine. Those that do seem to like it: seven out of ten who saw a chiropractor reported they were 'very satisfied', and six out of ten who went to an osteopath or acupuncturist said they were very pleased with their treatment.

Other non-conventional treatments are becoming more readily available. Every day, in health centres, community centres and private homes, men and women enjoy aromatherapy and reflexology. So many are treating themselves with herbal and homeopathic remedies that a leading chemist chain recently launched its own brand of products; 'rescue remedy' and arnica are now on the shelf next to paracetamol. Hostesses routinely offer their guests camomile tea to help them to relax, and citizens from 16 to 60 take vitamin and mineral supplements with their morning orange juice.

What is the difference between complementary medicine and alternative therapies?
Both these terms are generally applied to any form of treatment which is not generally provided by or taught to orthodox health care professionals such as doctors, dentists and nurses.

Complementary medicine is used to describe treatments which are generally used *alongside* orthodox medical treatment. Examples would include the professions of osteopathy and chiropractic, complementary therapies such as healing and shiatsu and self help measures such as yoga and T'ai chi chu'an. Practitioners usually expect patients to continue with any conventional medication or treatment that they have been prescribed.

Alternative therapies, on the other hand, is the term often used for treatments which are given *in place of* orthodox medical care. For example, herbal medicines may be prescribed by a medical herbalist in place of orthodox medical drugs.

Clearly there are circumstances when a complementary medicine can be used as an alternative to orthodox medicine, and occasions when an alternative medicine might be used in conjunction with orthodox medical treatment. Acupuncture, for example, can be an 'alternative' in treatment when it is used as part of the traditional Chinese system of medicine, whose whole approach to health is quite different from western medicine; but it is also frequently used as a form of complementary medicine by western doctors and other health care practitioners for the relief of pain.

Because of the confusion between the terms 'alternative' and 'complementary' medicine it is often easier to talk about 'non-conventional' medicine. What *is* common to both complementary and alternative forms of medicine is a 'holistic' philosophy of health. According to this view of health, physical sickness can affect our emotions, making us depressed or moody, and can even affect our inner spirit, that vital spark which makes us what we are. It works the other way too; negative feelings and emotions such as jealousy, anger and despair can affect and impair the function of our immune system, which fights disease, and leave us vulnerable to any passing bug.

Good health, therefore, is not simply a question of watching our blood pressure, exercising regularly and eating a balanced diet with plenty of fruit and vegetables. It is also about keeping the brain active, allowing our emotions natural expression, and approaching life with a positive attitude, seeking the best in ourselves and others. Ill health is seen as a lack of harmony in the way the body, mind and spirit work together. Treatment, therefore, must be aimed at mobilising the body's own healing mechanisms, which can then work to restore balance and health to the whole system.

Rather than treating a complaint like eczema, for example, as a symptom on its own with creams and lotions, the holistic practitioner will look for an underlying cause. What has thrown the system so out of balance that it triggers a skin reaction? It could be emotional, such as suppressed grief, or stress from over-work, the result of environmental pollution, an allergic response to food or a new washing powder.

According to the skills they practise, treatment from a complementary medical practitioner might include the prescription of a herbal remedy, or a particular diet to help cleanse the body and eliminate foods which may have provoked an allergic response. Touch, massage and aromatherapy oils are used to help ease tense muscles and reduce stress, or stimulate the acupuncture pressure points to improve the flow of 'Qi' energy around the body.

Of course, any orthodox doctor could use a holistic approach – and many do. Equally, some non-conventional practitioners may concentrate on specific symptoms.

Why is non-conventional medicine so popular?

Modern medical technology has made such quantum leaps that we have learnt to expect miracles, and it can be disappointing when the instant cure, the 'magic bullet', is not delivered. Yes, there are marvels: sight that is restored with laser surgery; life for babies born before time; spectacular triple bypass operations; heart swaps; kidney transplants. But there is still the nagging discomfort of arthritis, skin allergies, irritable bowel syndrome, back pain – chronic conditions that are so difficult to live with, and for which doctors still have no cure. Add to this the tarnished image of wonder drugs that fail to deal with the symptoms for which they are prescribed, or which replace them with risky and unpleasant side effects, combined with the arrogant and dismissive manner of some health professionals – 'We know what is best for your body. Don't ask so many questions and do as you are told' – and the disenchantment of so many patients begins to be understood. According to a 1993 survey in the *Daily Telegraph*, three out of four people visiting complementary practitioners went because of problems that orthodox medicine had failed to fix.

The current emphasis on preventive medicine – eat a healthy diet, take regular aerobic exercise, monitor yourself for lumps and bumps, learn stress-management techniques – encourages people to assume some control for their health, and they then expect to be involved when something goes wrong. Unfortunately, the amount of time, explanation and consultation that this demands is not, with the best will in the world, within the scope of the average GP. The move, therefore, to complementary medicine, with its emphasis on partnership, holism and healing powers, begins to seem natural in every sense.

Admittedly, there is little you can contribute to the technique of the acupuncturist or the osteopath's manipulation, but the very act of making an appointment somehow puts you in control. Once in the therapist's consulting room, there is usually a long and satisfying discussion, not just of your medical history, but about your eating and sleeping habits, likes and dislikes, your work and your relationships. Advice will often be given on suggested changes in lifestyle to improve and maintain health and fitness.

The physical touch that is so often involved is itself therapeutic. Osteopath, Caroline Penn, believes that the explosion of bodywork therapies is partly due to the stiff-upper-lip reserve of the British character:

'Our culture has been so physically standoffish that we have been starved of this kind of care for each other, and these therapies fulfil a real need.'

What do doctors think?

It is not just the lay public that is attracted to complementary treatments. About a third of GPs have some experience in one or more complementary treatments, and almost as many again are interested in training, especially women doctors and younger doctors.

This interest received a boost when, in 1991, Junior Health Minister, Stephen Dorrell, announced that GPs could recommend complementary medicine for their patients on the NHS, providing the doctor retained ultimate clinical responsibility.

Acupuncture, osteopathy, homeopathy and chiropractic are viewed most favourably by doctors, probably because they have an air of legitimacy. Osteopathy became a legally recognised profession, like dentistry, through an Act of Parliament in 1993, and chiropractic is expected to follow shortly. A number of GPs have studied acupuncture (though not necessarily to the level of non-medical acupuncturists) and practise it in NHS pain and addiction clinics. There are five NHS-run homeopathic hospitals in the UK, and increasing numbers of doctors are taking postgraduate training courses in homeopathy.

Nurses at NHS hospitals, such as the Royal Marsden and London's Hammersmith Hospital, are using 'touch' therapies to alleviate pain and encourage seriously ill and terminally ill patients to feel more positive. Only a few GPs and Family Health Service Authorities (FHSAs) are prepared to fund massage, aromatherapy and reflexology, but those who do find unexpected benefits.

Dr Sheila Hunt is a London GP who refers her stressed and anxiety-ridden patients to her practice nurse, who is trained in therapeutic massage:

> *'Being touched helps people unwind, so that patients open up with our nurse in a way they don't with me, and it becomes a counselling session.'*

Depending on whether they can afford it, and often to their surprise, she sometimes suggests that her patients consult the acupuncturist who practises next door. If they suffer from severe eczema, she might recommend the Chinese herbal doctor down the road:

> *'usually they have been through everything conventional medicine can offer and they're willing to try anything. Some would rather take herbs than a lengthy course of steroids. Occasionally I will suggest acupuncture as a first line treatment for PMS (premenstrual syndrome) if there is a wide range of symptoms that would need a variety of conventional medicines.'*

She has been impressed with the results:

> *'On the whole, people benefit because they appreciate something that treats them more as a whole person and not as a particular problem. We try to treat like that in the practice, but complementary practitioners can offer longer appointments – an hour or more compared to ten minutes.'*

Complementary medicine on the NHS?

Patients might say they want complementary medicine, and in theory it is available, but the reality appears different. On the one hand GPs seem unclear about how to obtain NHS funding for such treatments; on the other, District Health Authorities (DHAs) and fundholding doctors who control their own budgets need to be convinced of any savings and benefits.

Will complementary treatments cut the cost of drug bills or keep people out of hospital? Nobody really knows. The Alexander Technique for Mrs X could mean no chiropody for Mr Y. Where research does exist, it can be convincing. In a two-year study of over 700 people with chronic or severe back pain, chiropractic proved more effective than physiotherapy.

Barbara Connah of the National Association of Health Authorities and Trusts (NAHAT) states: 'Unless patients speak up we won't know what the demand is.' A recent poll showed that 80 per cent of people did not know it was possible to have complementary therapy on the NHS. She suggests that if your GP recommends tablets and rest for your bad back, enquire if osteopathy or chiropractic is available: 'Many patients assume it is not on offer, so they don't ask. But if enough did, then the GP or FHSA might be more willing to purchase it.'

Enough people were bypassing their GP and referring themselves to practitioners of non-conventional medicine, however, to prompt the British Medical Association (BMA) to look into the situation. Its report, *Complementary medicine, new approaches to good practice*, was published in 1993.

The BMA stated that if such a demand existed, then it was important the public be assured of receiving competent and responsible treatment: doctors should find out more about complementary therapies in order to advise their patients, so they should attend courses that explained which were the most popular and beneficial.

One of the best ways of finding out about non-conventional practitioners is to work alongside them. Dr Patrick Pietroni founded the pioneering Marylebone Health Centre in London seven years ago, an NHS practice with complementary therapists on site. Others followed – Dr George Lewith's Centre for the Study of Complementary Medicine in Southampton, the Hale Clinic in London – but they are largely private. A few fundholding GPs will refer patients to complementary practitioners, and some even employ non-conventional practitioners or rent them space to practise within their surgery.

Such a relationship is not always a comfortable one. Patients are seen by a doctor, who may then refer them to a practitioner – but which one? An acupuncturist? A hypnotherapist? And for which disorders? Someone has to take the decisions, and professional jealousy can arise.

Dr David Peters is a homeopath and osteopath who trained as a doctor and works at the Marylebone Health Centre. He believes that the people GPs tend to refer to complementary therapists are those they cannot cure – 'difficult' patients who are chronically sick or depressed, for whom complementary medicine may offer the most help.

Does complementary medicine work?

There is an overwhelming need for information about complementary medicine, not only among doctors but also patients. What does the therapist actually do? Do the treatments work? Do the therapists know what they are doing?

Patients may say they feel better, but the fact is that very little research has been done into non-conventional therapy. There are various reasons for this, one being a lack of money.

Pharmaceutical companies spend vast sums on the manufacture and testing of synthetic drug products that could yield even vaster profits. Few non-conventional therapies involve medication and, even where they do – as with herbal and homeopathic remedies –

the manufacturers are small companies who simply do not have funds for the kind of large-scale testing required to label their products as medicines.

Another reason for the lack of research is that non-conventional medicine is so different, so subjective, so *sensitive* compared to orthodox treatments that some people claim they cannot be investigated in the same way. There may be an element of truth in this, but critics insist that randomised, double-blind clinical trials – the backbone of scientific research – could still be applied to many therapies.

However, until such rigorous research is done, sceptics will argue that patients would have got better anyway, or that any improvement is due to what is called the 'placebo' effect. This is an accepted phenomenon in which the patient's belief in the treatment, or faith in the practitioner, is so powerful that, in as many as three out of ten cases, it works. The placebo effect has been known, among other things, to reduce blood pressure, heal ulcers, reduce swelling, override the effects of stimulants and relieve arthritis, hayfever and depression. Scientific trials always make allowances for it, and it probably deserves more research in its own right.

Only when clinical trials show results above that of the placebo are they taken seriously. At least two studies of homeopathic remedies have achieved this, those for arthritis and hayfever, at Glasgow University and Glasgow Homeopathic Hospital. The Centre for Complementary Studies at Exeter University has several projects under way, and the Research Council for Complementary Medicine (RCCM) is an independent charity that provides advice and support for research. Such research and experiments are costly and funds are desperately needed.

On another level, scientists are asking *why* complementary medicine and alternative therapies work. Interest is focusing on a new field of study called psychoneuroimmunology (PNI). This looks into the links between psychology, neurophysiology and immunology – the mind–body connection that holistic therapists have always believed in. Leading-edge research in the US indicates that stress and loneliness are risk factors for diseases of all kinds, from the common cold to AIDS, and there is evidence that our emotions may trigger biochemical responses which affect the immune system.

Is the practitioner competent?

What patients ask, and doctors need to know, is how to find a competent practitioner. If doctors refer patients to complementary practitioners, they are still responsible for the health of those patients. If patients refer themselves to a practitioner they should feel confident that any undiagnosed serious condition will be recognised and they will be advised to seek appropriate help.

Dr George Lewith of the Centre for the Study of Complementary Medicine, Southampton, states:

> *'Competence means different things to different people. If you want a competent aromatherapist who will massage you for an hour so that you feel good, that is one thing, but a non-medically qualified acupuncturist claiming a complete diagnostic system is another. If you do not know what is wrong with you, don't go to someone who hasn't the skill to make a medical diagnosis.'*

This is a serious and controversial issue. The BMA Report describes the professions of acupuncture, homeopathy, osteopathy, herbal medicine and chiropractic as 'discrete, clinical disciplines', distinguished from other forms of non-conventional medicine by having more established foundations of training, clinical practice and professional standards. Because they involve the use of either physical manipulation or invasive techniques (you either swallow something or have needles inserted into you), they have the potential, in untrained hands, to do harm as well as good.

It is important, therefore, that practitioners of these 'discrete, clinical disciplines' are properly trained and regulated by an appropriate professional body. Qualified osteopaths and chiropractors, for example, undergo a clinical training which is grounded in the orthodox medical sciences. They are trained to be aware of their limits of competence and to know when a patient is suffering from a condition which requires referral to a GP. 'If I had raging pneumonia, I wouldn't mess around sticking needles in myself,' remarked one acupuncturist.

Some doctors take courses in acupuncture and homeopathy in addition to their medical training, but the extent of these courses has been criticised. There is also real concern that some lay acupuncturists and homeopaths insist on making diagnoses outside the conventional system.

One doctor recalls:

'The daughter of a friend of mine was suffering from a raging middle ear infection that would make her deaf if she was not put on a course of antibiotics, yet she had been taken for weeks to a homeopath, who fiddled about prescribing one remedy after another. The man had not even looked into the child's ear.'

Although acupuncturists and homeopaths object to such accusations, cases like this underline the BMA's concern about possible risks. It believes that these 'discrete, clinical disciplines' should be legally regulated, and this requires an Act of Parliament, something the osteopaths achieved in 1993. A new governing body, the General Osteopathic Council (GOsC), will establish and maintain minimum standards of training, and enforce a code of professional conduct. No one will be entitled to be called an osteopath who is not on the Council's register of qualified practitioners. Without such regulation, anybody can do a weekend training course, put a few letters after their name, and call themselves a hypnotherapist, a herbalist, or whatever they choose. The public has no protection against either charlatans or bunglers.

A number of EU countries take a tougher line on this situation, and so when British joined the Common Market, many therapies were nudged into 'getting their act together', as they put it, and setting their own standards of practice.

The BMA regards therapies such as massage and reflexology as less of a potential hazard than the 'discrete, clinical disciplines,' and believes that voluntary systems of regulation can provide patients with adequate safeguards providing the professions concerned adopt a code of conduct, proper training structures and a voluntary register of members.

There is also consumer pressure. As people become more informed about complementary medicine, they become more discerning. They expect therapists to know what they are doing, and they are more ready to complain if anything goes wrong.

Standards vary enormously. Training, for example, can vary from three or four weekends in some cases to a four or five year full-time degree course in others. NVQs (national vocational qualifications) are currently being investigated as indicators of competence that everyone can recognise.

There is a MSc course for qualified osteopaths offered by the European School of Osteopathy.

Honours degree courses are now available in osteopathy and chiropractic and a BSc in medical herbalism is in the final stages of discussion. Exeter University offers a B.Phil in Complementary Health studies, and the University of Westminster has launched postgraduate MAs in therapeutic bodywork and holistic healthcare.

How to choose a practitioner

Why you want to try complementary medicine is an important question to consider, as it may affect your choice both of treatment and practitioner. Do you want to try it to enhance your overall well-being, or do you have a specific health problem which has been diagnosed by a conventional doctor? Are you receiving orthodox treatment, or have you already tried it and found it inadequate?

When it comes to finding a qualified practitioner, your GP may be as confused as you are. Many people choose a practitioner by word of mouth, which may be reassuring but not infallible. If you are referring yourself to complementary medicine, you owe it to yourself to make sure the practitioner is adequately trained and reputable.

Ask yourself and the practitioner the following questions. They are based on an excellent consumer checklist drawn up by the Royal College of Nursing, and includes suggestions from the BMA.

- What are the practitioner's qualifications? What sort of training was undertaken and for how long?

- How many years has the practitioner been in practice?

- Is the practitioner registered with a recognised organisation, and does this organisation have:
  - a public register?
  - a code of practice, specifying the professional conduct required?
  - an effective disciplinary procedure and sanctions?
  - a complaints system?

- Can the practitioner give you the address and telephone number of this organisation?

- Is the therapy available on the NHS?

- Can the GP delegate your care to the practitioner?

- Is this the most appropriate complementary treatment for your problem?

- What does the treatment actually involve? What will you be expected to do?

- Does the practitioner send a letter to your GP advising of any treatment received?

- What is the practitioner's attitude to any orthodox medicine you may be receiving?

- Can you claim for the treatment through your private health insurance scheme, if you have one?

- Are your records confidential?

- What is the cost of the treatment?

- How many treatments should you expect to need, and what will be the approximate overall cost?

- Is the practitioner covered by professional indemnity insurance, so that you can receive compensation if the practitioner is found to be negligent?

After your initial consultation, ask yourself these questions.

- Did the practitioner answer your questions clearly and to your satisfaction?

- Did the practitioner conduct her/himself in a professional manner?

- Were you given information to look through at your leisure?

- Is the practitioner making excessive claims about the treatment?

Avoid any practitioner

- who claims to cure your illness. No form of treatment, conventional or complementary, is perfect. Most non-conventional treatments assist in the healing process. Some may work for you, but miracles should not be expected.

- who suggests you throw out your conventional medicine without first consulting your doctor.

- with whom you feel uncomfortable. Consultations with practitioners of complementary medicine are usually conducted on a one-to-one basis, and may involve removing clothes as well as touch. An important factor in healing is also the rapport you establish with the practitioner, who should encourage you to take responsibility for your own well-being.

For further information, see *Finding a qualified practitioner* (page 143) which lists professional organisations and registering bodies for each treatment.

A–Z OF COMPLEMENTARY MEDICINES AND THERAPIES

At a rough estimate, there are well over a hundred complementary therapies in practice in Britain, and more surface almost daily. Fascinating as they all are, in this book we can only attempt to deal with the better known and more widely available.

Rating the therapies

How popular is a therapy with the public? What do doctors think of it? Is there scientific evidence that it works? How easy is it to find a practitioner?

The complementary therapies have been rated according to popularity, medical credibility, scientific research, and availability by Dr David Peters, homeopath, osteopath and general practitioner, chair of the British Holistic Medical Association, and Course Director of the Centre for Community Care and Primary Health, University of Westminster.

Key to symbols

Popularity	*	obscure
	**	has a following
	***	up and coming
	****	in demand
Medical credibility	*	antagonism
	**	indifference
	***	interest
	****	acceptance
Scientific research	*	non-existent
	**	anecdotal
	***	some studies
	****	in the best journals
Availability	*	almost invisible
	**	scattered
	***	growing
	****	widespread

ACUPRESSURE

Described as acupuncture without the needles, this may have been oriental doctors' first method of treatment some 3000 years ago when they mapped the meridian system (see *Acupuncture*). The practitioner presses specific points on the body with the fingers and thumbs to stimulate and restore the flow of the life energy force (Qi). One form is closer to *shiatsu*, and employs elbows and knees for extra pressure. Another, Shen Tao, uses fingers only and lighter pressure to tap more subtle energy patterns.

Best for
Acupressure claims to relieve (though not cure) allergies, arthritis, asthma, backache, circulation problems, constipation, depression, digestive problems, high blood pressure, insomnia, muscular tension, migraine, nausea, premenstrual syndrome (PMS), skin disorders, and water retention.

What happens
A practitioner begins with a detailed consultation, exploring your medical and family history, diet, and way of life. You sit or lie on a treatment table or the floor. No equipment or oils are used and, although it is not necessary to undress, it is a good idea to wear loose-fitting clothes. The experience feels like a firm massage and can be very relaxing and revitalising. Because it is simple and non-invasive, side effects are rare.

Self-help
You can practise basic acupressure techniques on yourself. For example, pressing the web of flesh between thumb and forefinger on one hand with your other thumb and forefinger activates a pressure point that relieves headache, toothache, cramps and constipation.

Doctors say
A stimulating massage of any kind will help produce endorphins, the body's pain-relieving hormones. Also, according to the 'gate control theory' of pain relief, nerves carrying pressure messages reach the brain faster than pain messages and will close the 'gate', as the brain can only receive so many messages at once.

Research at Belfast University found that acupressure bands which press a meridian point on the wrist, could relieve nausea caused by general anaesthesia, pregnancy, travel sickness and some drugs.

Rating

Popularity	Medical Credibility	Scientific Research	Availability
✭✭	✭✭	✭✭	✭✭✭

ACUPUNCTURE

Practitioners of this ancient oriental system of healing insert needles into specific points of the body in order to restore the balance of Qi energy considered essential for good health. Its origin is lost in the mists of time, but allegedly the practice began when soldiers surviving arrow wounds found they also recovered from long-standing complaints.

According to traditional Chinese medicine, Qi (pronounced chee) is the universal life energy that is concentrated in our bodies along invisible channels beneath the skin called meridians. There are said to be 14 main meridian channels that run to and from the hands and feet to the body and head, and along these are dotted the acupuncture points where Qi enters and exits the body. Traditional practitioners identified only 365 of these, but modern acupuncturists now work with up to 2000.

Qi is activated by the constant movement of energy between two opposite and complementary qualities known as the Yin and the Yang. It is a delicate balance that can be upset by a number of factors, found in abundance in Western living, including infections, poisons and accidents that cause physical ailments; emotional states such as stress, anger or grief; spiritual neglect; poor diet (too much sweet, salty, greasy or spicy food, rushed and erratic meals); drugs (whether prescribed or recreational); weather conditions and genetic inheritance.

Yang and Yin correspond roughly to our concepts of male and female, active and passive, expanding and contracting, hollow and solid, positive and negative, light and dark. Yin organs are dense and blood-filled, such as the heart and liver. Dull aches and pains, chilliness, fluid retention, and fatigue are often due to excess yin. Yang organs are those involved with discharge or absorption, such as the gall bladder and stomach. Too much yang can be expressed as acute pain, inflammation, spasms, headache and high blood pressure.

When Yin and Yang are out of balance, the flow of Qi energy is interrupted and we are susceptible to disease and emotional disorder. Stimulating the key points with needles (acupuncture), pressure (*acupressure, shiatsu*), heat (burning small bundles of moxa herb over the area, a process called moxibustion), cupping (inverting glass cups to create a vacuum and increase blood supply), mild electrical currents, or lasers (popular with conventional doctors) can free the flow of Qi where there is a blockage, or restore it to depleted areas, thus bringing the body into harmony again.

Best for

Those suffering anxiety, arthritis, asthma, depression, problems with circulation, fatigue, hay fever, headaches, high blood pressure, intestinal problems, musculo-skeletal problems, painful periods, PMS. Some people have found it helpful for ME (myalgic encephalomayelitis) and menopausal symptoms. It is increasingly considered in pregnancy and it works well for children when explained carefully.

What happens

At the first visit, the acupuncturist takes detailed notes of your symptoms, medical and family history, lifestyle and diet. He or she will want to know whether your bowels move regularly, if you sleep soundly, feel anxious or are quick to row with your partner. Appearance and behaviour will be studied: the tone of your skin and hair, how you move, the way you speak, what gestures you make. As part of the traditional Chinese diagnosis, your tongue will be examined for structure, colour and coating, and a check made of the 12 meridian pulses, six on each wrist, for quality, rhythm and strength. All this is to build up a total picture that will guide the diagnosis and choice of treatment.

Acupuncture needles are of fine stainless steel and insertion is quick and, allegedly, painless and bloodless, although a slight ache or tingle known as the 'needle sensation' may be felt when they are in place. They may remain for a few minutes or for half an hour, depending on the condition being treated and your reaction. Acupuncturists usually insert the needles just below the skin to a depth of about a quarter to half an inch, depending on where they are in the body. Chinese acupuncturists may on occasion insert them slightly deeper. As a general rule, the more experienced the practitioner, the fewer needles used.

Treatment sessions usually cost from £30–£35 for the initial visit and often less thereafter. They usually last 30 to 90 minutes, once or twice a week, but there is no set number. If the effects are dramatic, only one or two sessions may be required; sometimes it is a more subtle process that takes months. However, some change should be expected after five treatments.

People are rightly anxious about the risk of contracting HIV from an infected needle. Boiling is not enough, and it is important to consult a practitioner who is also a qualified doctor or is accredited by one of the five member bodies of the Council for Acupuncture, who follow strict rules about hygiene and sterilisation of equipment in an autoclave. Many acupuncturists now use disposable needles, so ask for these if you are concerned.

Jo, a graphic designer in her 20s, spoke of her experience:

'Initially I went to an acupuncturist because I wanted something to buck me up and give me more energy. The nagging neck and back pain I had seemed a side thing. The acupuncturist is Chinese and has rooms in the same centre as my NHS GP, so I just made an appointment. The first time I went, he was comforting and reassuring and felt my back and said "You've got ankylosing spondylitis", a kind of arthritis in the back which my sister suffers from and is hereditary, so instantly I was convinced by him.

'The first treatment lasted half an hour, and when I left I felt ten

inches taller, and more alive and energised than I had for ages.
When I got home, my boyfriend said "Gosh, you look well!"
which has inspired me to keep going back.

'He inserts four needles, four inches deep, just above the base
of the spine, and another eight up my back, neck and shoulders,
then puts a very gentle electrical current through them and leaves
them for about twenty minutes. It's not that painful when the
needles go in, but the current throbs and is a bit uncomfortable –
I feel like a laboratory frog wired up to electrodes. A couple of
times it did bleed a little, accidentally, but I can feel it doing me
good, pulsing away, dissipating my pain. You undress as much
as is necessary – I take off my bra and lie face down on the
treatment table, and I have never felt awkward.

'I've been going now for two years, every two weeks, at £25 a
go, which I'm prepared to pay but I wish it could be on the NHS.
I let it slip for a few months once, but the neck pains came back
even worse, and I've realised it's worth keeping up now, and
I still feel brighter and more alert after each treatment.'

Doctors say

GPs are increasingly referring patients to acupuncturists, as people
report the benefits of treatment. It is always advisable to check
symptoms with your doctor first, in case they are due to serious
conditions, such as cancer, which a lay acupuncturist might miss.

Acupuncture is not generally available on the NHS, although a
number of pain clinics attached to major hospitals use acupuncture
for pain relief. Its effectiveness here is attributed to its ability to
prevent pain signals reaching the brain before the 'gate' is closed
(see p.15). Research also shows that acupuncture releases
endorphins and enkephalins, the body's pain-killing hormones,
into the nervous system.

Nobody has yet come up with scientific evidence of the meridian
system (which orthodox medicine finds difficult to accept), but
acupuncture points have been shown to have a lower electrical
resistance than surrounding skin.

Rating

Popularity	Medical Credibility	Scientific Research	Availability
✮✮✮✮	✮✮✮✮	✮✮✮✮	✮✮✮✮

ALEXANDER TECHNIQUE

The Alexander Technique teaches you to improve your posture so that you stand and move more efficiently and gracefully, as humans were designed to do, without straining your body. In this sense, it is not really a therapy; practitioners call themselves teachers, and have pupils or students, not patients or clients. But people who have learnt the Technique say that not only do they feel in better health, but physical disorders improve and their mental alertness and emotional well-being are enhanced. It seems to be a clear example of the interconnection of mind and body, and the knock-on effect that treating one has upon the other.

As babies and small children we possess a natural poise, but, as we grow older and spend hours hunched at a desk, our bodies become twisted and enormous stress is placed on our skeleton and muscles. Our joints stiffen, breathing is shallow, circulation impaired, the spine curves, and aches and pains appear. Bad posture often goes hand in hand with psychological problems – those suffering from depression tend to stoop and collapse down on themselves, compared to the upright stance of a confident person.

We become so accustomed to a lifetime's bad habits that we no longer know what we are doing wrong, and have to be taught the correct way to hold ourselves – which is what teachers of the Alexander Technique do.

One teacher said:

> *'When the phone rings, people tend to become tense and rush to pick it up, rather than calmly strolling over to it. Most people use far more pressure than necessary just to open a door or turn on a tap, but usually they don't realise it. An Alexander teacher*

*will make them aware of this. They take the pupil through
a movement, monitor how much tension they are putting into
it and then tell them how they can do it with less effort.'*

When Frederick Matthias Alexander, an Australian actor in the late nineteenth century, began to lose his voice, there seemed to be no medical explanation. Studying himself in the mirror, he discovered that, before he spoke, he pulled back his head and the muscles in his throat visibly tightened. By counteracting these constrictions he restored his voice, found that his physical and mental health improved, and went on to develop his theory that lengthening the neck muscles frees the spine and empowers the body. He moved to London, where grateful students included George Bernard Shaw, Aldous Huxley and a host of actors and musicians, and in 1931 he set up the first training school for teachers of what was now called the Alexander Technique.

Best for
Learning the technique can offer relief from anxiety, arthritis, asthma, lower back pain, depression, fatigue, stiff neck or shoulders, peptic ulcers, high blood pressure, irritable bowel syndrome, repetitive strain injury (RSI), respiratory disorders, sciatica, stress and tension headaches. Epileptics say it can reduce their number of seizures, and it may alleviate many gynaecological disorders, including heavy periods.

What happens
Alexander Technique teachers usually work one-to-one with their pupils/students. In the first lesson, the teacher assesses the way you stand and move. While you sit or lie down, he or she uses gentle manipulation – subtle hand movements and pressures – to make you aware of problem areas and let you know what optimum body posture feels like. 'People step off my couch two inches taller,' says Gwyneth, who has taught the technique for twenty years. 'They go out looking like kings and queens.'

A full course consists of anything from 15 to 30 half-hour to three-quarter hour sessions, depending on how well you pick it up and how frequently you can go (twice a week is recommended), and costs from £13–£40 per session. The teacher re-educates your way of standing, moving, sitting down, standing up, lying down, walking and lifting objects, and you will be expected to put in some practice between classes. No special clothes are necessary, but wear something loose-fitting.

Jane, a 42-year-old English teacher with two children, learnt the Alexander Technique because:

'my shoulders ached with tension, I felt exhausted, and I knew my posture was dreadful: one hip was higher than the other, from carrying heavy briefcases, babies and baskets of laundry. The best bit of the lessons was lying on the couch while the teacher arranged my body how it should be, which felt wonderful. The hardest bit was trying to attain that degree of grace on your own!

'You learn what are called the 'orders' which you repeat until they become automatic and your body is programmed to follow them. Free the neck. Think of the head going forward and up. Allow the back to lengthen and widen. Even thinking of them makes me feel taller and more co-ordinated.

'I had about 15 classes, at the end of which not only had my hips levelled, but I developed a more balanced sense of priorities. I realised my life was unnecessarily stressful, and I resigned from several committees that ate up too much of my time.'

Doctors say

Doctors' attitudes to the Alexander Technique are almost universally benign, and many GPs recommend a course to their patients, probably because there is little in what it teaches that conflicts with medical practice. It does no harm and will probably do some good.

Scientific studies show that the technique is good for breathing, improving muscular and respiratory function. Recent research in London confirms its value in relieving back pain.

Rating

Popularity	Medical Credibility	Scientific Research	Availability
✫✫✫	✫✫✫	✫✫✫	✫✫✫

ANTHROPOSOPHICAL MEDICINE

More of an alternative attitude to health and sickness than a therapy, anthroposophical medicine is based on the philosophy of the Austrian scientist, Rudolf Steiner.

Steiner taught that, as well as a physical body, humans have an 'etheric' body that encourages growth; an 'astral' body governing the senses and emotions; and an 'ego', the spiritual consciousness of oneself. All these systems should be in balance for perfect health, but, because of our need to grow and develop, this balance is always changing. Although Christian in outlook, anthroposophy believes in reincarnation and that our health in this life reflects the 'karma' or load carried from past lives.

Practitioners must qualify as orthodox doctors first. Although popular in Europe, where there are hundreds of doctors and several hospitals, anthroposophical medicine has had rather a lean time in the UK, until the current interest in complementary therapies. It has been hard for students to reconcile modern medicine's reliance on pharmaceuticals and surgery with anthroposophy's preference for natural remedies. Before, or as well as, using conventional methods, an anthroposophical doctor might prescribe homoeopathic and herbal remedies, special massage, hydrotherapy, art therapy, music and speech therapy, counselling and curative eurhythmy, in which movement is linked to speech and music.

Rating

Popularity	Medical Credibility	Scientific Research	Availability
✫✫	✫✫	✫✫✫	✫✫

AROMATHERAPY

Nothing irritates an aromatherapist more than hearing the description 'massage with smells' – although this is often how most people experience a treatment now considered the most popular of all complementary therapies.

Massage might be a particularly agreeable way of applying aromatic and therapeutic essential plant oils, and one that more and more nurses, midwives and health visitors are learning to use – touch is a powerful therapy in itself – but it is only one means of delivering the powerful molecules of the oils to the nervous and circulatory systems of the body and the olfactory centres of the brain. They can also be inhaled, added to baths, used as a compress, or (more rarely) swallowed.

Essential oils are usually extracted from plants by distillation. The plant essence is heated until it vaporises in steam and, when cooled, separates into water and the essential oil.

An oil may come from the leaves, as in eucalyptus, another from the roots, such as ginger, and particular therapeutic properties are claimed for each. Lavender, tea-tree and geranium, for instance, are known to be efficient fighters of infections caused (in corresponding order) by bacteria, fungi and viruses.

Neroli is derived from the flowers of the bitter orange tree. This oil has a refreshing and revivifying aroma, and calming and comforting qualities for those suffering from shock, stress-related conditions and palpitations. Aromatherapists use it for nervous diarrhoea, indigestion and insomnia, and sometimes for scarring and broken veins. Lovers claim it heightens sexual arousal, and it has long been associated with fertility – one reason that brides traditionally wear orange blossom in their hair.

The medicinal properties of plant oils have been recognised for thousands of years. The ancient Persians, Egyptians (who put them to good use in embalming), Greeks and Arabs all employed them. The work of the eleventh century physician and philosopher Ali ibn Sina (known in the West as Avicenna), who studied the effects of more than 800 plants, was brought back to Europe by the Crusaders.

In the Middle Ages and the Elizabethan period, aromatic oils were popular as medicines and perfumes (particularly as bathing was viewed with suspicion), but manufacturers began taking short cuts in production, and they lost their reputation for efficacy.

It was in the 1920s, when a French chemist, René-Maurice Gattefosse, accidentally burnt his hand while working in the family perfume house and applied lavender oil to soothe the burn, that aromatherapy as we know it made an appearance. Gattefosse's hand healed more quickly than expected and with less scarring. Intrigued, he made a study of the therapeutic qualities of plant oils.

His work was picked up in the 1960s by Marguerite Maury, also French, a biochemist and beautician, who was more interested in the rejuvenating virtues of essential oils and wrote a book, *The Secret of Life and Youth*. Meanwhile, another Frenchman, Dr Jean Valnet, claimed to have successfully used oils in treating burns, cancer, diabetes, TB and other physical and emotional disturbances.

Aromatherapy initially gained popularity in the UK as a kind of beauty treatment, and it is only relatively recently that health professionals have begun to take its healing potential seriously. Quite how smell can affect the brain, our moods and ultimately our health is still something of a mystery, although it is known that lavender appears to increase alpha brain rhythms, typical of a relaxed state, and that jasmine triggers beta rhythms, associated with alertness.

Some substances are absorbed into the bloodstream through the skin, as in massage. Others are inhaled into the nose and lungs, either by hanging over a bowl of very hot water to which a few drops of oil have been added, or, less effectively though more deliciously, by soaking in a bath.

Essential oils are complex chemicals, and it is suspected that, once on the body, their nature changes. Pheromones, hormones secreted by all animals including humans, cannot be consciously detected, and yet they have powerful effects on behaviour. Why, for instance, should we find one person sexually attractive and not another? The infinitely more obvious scent of essential oils could well work in a similar way.

Best for

According to the International Federation of Aromatherapists (IFA), aromatherapy 'enhances well-being, relieves stress, and helps in the rejuvenation and regeneration of the human body.' More specifically, it has been used to treat stress-related conditions, such as depression, anger, anxiety and insomnia; skin conditions, such as acne and eczema; digestive disorders including diarrhoea and constipation; and minor infections, such as cystitis. Pain, arthritis and cramp have also responded to massage with essential oils.

What happens

At your first appointment, the aromatherapist will spend half an hour or so asking questions about your diet, exercise, posture, skin, sleeping patterns, moods and general health and medical history. Then she or he will choose two or more essential oils that will enhance your mood and alleviate your health problems.

These chosen oils are blended and diluted in a carrier oil, lotion or cream for massage. An aromatherapy massage is based on Swedish massage, aimed at relieving tension, draining lymph fluid and improving circulation so that the oils can circulate through the body. A back massage – for which you remove all clothes above the waist – takes about half an hour; a full body massage lasts about 90 minutes. Sessions cost from £20 to £35, with massage.

Vivienne, a 34-year-old teacher with two young children, says:

> *'Someone said that aromatherapy might help the premenstrual tension that turns me into a monster every month. Before doing anything, Marian asked me a lot of questions about what I ate, how many hours I worked, whether I enjoyed my job, if my periods were painful, etcetera, etcetera. I undressed and hopped up on the couch and she covered me with towels. From her impressive collection of little bottles she chose three oils, rose, geranium and clary sage, that she thought would help my mood and hormonal state, and mixed them together with what she called a carrier oil – she used sweet almond.*

> *'The mixture smelt wonderful. She said the effects could be more overwhelming than I probably anticipated, and advised me not*

to drive home afterwards. She massaged my face and shoulders, then my back, arms, legs, and – very gently – my tummy, only uncovering the bits she was working on so that I wouldn't get cold. It was 90 minutes of utter, absolute bliss. When she finished I was nearly asleep and could hardly move. She was right about the impact; I got a taxi home and collapsed into bed for the rest of the afternoon.

'*On Marion's suggestion, I bought these essential oils, and a week before my period I'll add six to eight drops of each to my bath. Or, before going to bed, I might put ten drops each of clary sage and geranium and five of rose in 25 mls of carrier oil and massage myself, though not nearly as thoroughly as she did. I can't say that it has cured my PMS, as I still get very ratty, but I do feel more relaxed after using the oils.*'

Self-help

The more popular essential oils are easily available from health shops. Add six to eight drops to a warm bath and relax for at least ten minutes. To inhale, put six to ten drops on a tissue and take deep breaths, or add them to a bowl of steaming hot water. Never inhale directly from the bottle. For a massage, use 15 drops to 50 ml of carrier oil, and either apply it yourself, or ask a friend or partner.

Warning

Because they smell nice and are used in beauty treatments, people tend to forget that essential plant oils are not just perfumes. They are powerful substances and can be toxic. Never use them neat on the skin (apart from lavender and tea-tree oil, in emergencies). If you are pregnant, epileptic or suffer from high blood pressure, *always* consult a qualified aromatherapist first. Keep them away from children and out of the eyes. *Never* swallow any oils unless you are under the supervision of a trained aromatherapist.

Always buy high quality essential oils. Some of the products claiming to be essential oils are synthetic or diluted, and will not be effective. The Aromatherapy Trade Council (ATC), which has been formed to raise the standards of quality and safety, recommends that you only buy oils in dark glass bottles which have integral droppers in their necks. They should have clear instructions and contraindications, if not on the bottle then on the accompanying leaflet.

Doctors say

Although doctors are becoming more interested and increasing numbers of nurses are learning aromatherapy, it is only recently that serious research has begun. Peppermint oil has proved successful in clinical trials for irritable bowel syndrome, and tea-tree and lavender oil have been found effective in wound healing. A particular lavender oil reduced postoperative stress in heart patients in a study at the Bristol Royal Infirmary.

Rating

Popularity	Medical Credibility	Scientific Research	Availability
✫✫✫✫	✫✫✫	✫✫✫	✫✫✫✫

ART THERAPY

Expressing one's innermost feelings through painting, drawing, sculpting and modelling can help people bypass conscious thought, and articulate inaccessible emotions like rage or grief in a non-verbal way. Not only is it intensely satisfying for the patient, but the experience can mobilise their own healing powers.

In mainstream medicine, art therapy is used by psychiatrists and psychotherapists as supplementary treatment, to help diagnose and monitor a patient's condition. However, many otherwise healthy people who are suffering emotional distress, such as a bereavement, have found that spontaneous expression through paints and crayons is extremely therapeutic. Being 'good at art' is not a prerequisite!

Best for

Those suffering from drug and alcohol addiction and eating disorders and people who have difficulty communicating feelings with others benefit from this form of therapy.

Doctors say

Although theirs is a relatively new therapy, art therapists are now recognised and accepted in many NHS psychiatric hospital wards.

Rating

Popularity	Medical Credibility	Scientific Research	Availability
✮✮✮	✮✮✮	✮✮✮	✮✮✮✮

AURA HEALING (see HEALING)

The aura is described as a field of energy – possibly electromagnetic – around the body, the colours and brightness of which reflect our state of physical, emotional and spiritual health.

AUTOGENIC TRAINING

Businessmen in suits and airline pilots happily learn autogenic training, because it is presented as a sensible scientific way to programme yourself to relax at will. Dr Malcolm Carruthers brought the system to the UK in the 1970s, after encountering it in Canada where it was based on the 1930s research of German psychiatrist, Johannes Schultz.

Dr Carruthers describes it as 'a series of easy mental exercises designed to switch off the stress "fight or flight" system of the body, and switch on the "rest, relaxation and recreation" system.' The method is a process similar to self-hypnosis, yoga and meditation.

Best for

People suffering from stress-related symptoms such as migraine, eczema, high blood pressure, palpitations, irritable bowel syndrome, indigestion, colitis, ulcers, anxiety, tiredness, insomnia, depression, nervous tension and PMS, as well as people with AIDS, bronchitis and those trying to overcome an addiction, could benefit from using this technique.

What happens

Like the Alexander Technique, once you have learnt the method, you continue practising on your own. Courses are usually ninety-minute classes, once a week for eight weeks, in groups of six or eight students, at a hospital or private clinic. When you apply, you will be asked to fill in a form with details of your medical and mental history, and interviewed to make sure that you are physically and psychologically suitable. Those suffering heart conditions, for example, might be advised to learn under medical supervision; or diabetics and pregnant women might follow a modified version.

No special equipment or clothes are needed; the system is taught sitting or lying down. Eventually you will be adept enough to switch into it wherever you happen to be – even standing in a crowded commuter train.

Autogenic training consists of six basic exercises aimed at inducing profound and healing relaxation: feelings of heaviness ('my right arm is heavy'); warmth ('my left leg is warm'); concentration on the heartbeat; calming the breath; warmth in the stomach; coolness on the forehead. Each instruction is visualised (your *heavy* arm is made of *lead*) and repeated three times.

Dr Carruthers compares the system to driving a car in three phases. At the start you get into a comfortable position behind the wheel; then you change gear from your everyday state of mind to what he calls 'passive concentration'. Stopping – getting ready to return to ordinary stressful life – is important: you open your eyes, clench fists, bend arms, and then stretch your arms up and yawn, concentrating on feeling heaviness and warmth in different parts of the body.

Between classes, in which you compare notes on progress with other students, you are expected to practise at home, increasing from two or three minutes to 15 to 20 minutes three times a day, keeping a detailed diary of your responses. Some who have studied the method say it is not as easy to learn as one might think, and – like most things – works better for some than for others. A number of people, rather to their disconcertment, find themselves crying or laughing – or both – as repressed emotions are released.

Philip, a 39-year-old administrator, says:

'Autogenic training wasn't difficult to learn, but it did require a determined effort to set aside the time to practise. I found it fairly similar to other relaxation and meditation techniques, but it is more systematic and certainly more acceptable for the average Westerner who is wary of bells and mysticism, especially as classes are held in clinical surroundings.

'I really do find it useful in combating stress, and it definitely sharpened my powers of concentration. They suggest you leave little coloured dots around your office furniture as visual reminders to apply the techniques. I put one on the front of my boss's desk. He never noticed.'

Once the basics are mastered, you can move on to autogenic modification, which concentrates on specific areas (an asthma sufferer might say 'my sinuses are cool and my chest is warm'); to behaviour control, to help release writer's block or heighten athletic performance; and, finally, to autogenic meditation, to enable contact with your deepest levels of being.

Doctors say

There is considerable research to support the claim that autogenic training is an effective method of reducing stress. Orthodox doctors, health professionals and conventional people feel comfortable because it is objective, straightforward and makes no claim to a quasi-spiritual philosophy.

Rating

Popularity	Medical Credibility	Scientific Research	Availability
✫✫✫	✫✫✫	✫✫✫	✫✫✫

AYURVEDIC MEDICINE

Ayurveda, from the Sanskrit 'The Science of Life', is the ancient holistic healing system of India, derived from the Vedas and nearly 3000 years old. Although less well-known in the West, it is considered as sophisticated and comprehensive as the increasingly popular traditional Chinese medicine. Ayurvedic texts, as early as the fifth century BC, referred to surgery with primitive endoscopes and the body as composed of cells, 2000 years before the microscope was invented.

Like Chinese medicine, the underlying philosophy is that of balance between active energies. There are five basic elements or *doshas*: earth (solid components of the body, like bones); water (fluids and soft tissue); fire (heat, digestion and biochemical processes); air (sensation, the nervous system); and ether (networks and channels). The three basic energetic qualities or *gunas* are sattva (wise, unifying); rajas (active, creating, comparable with the Chinese yang) and tamas (passive, comparable with yin).

Best for
As a complete guide for physical health, well-being and spiritual energy, ayurveda claims to treat all diseases found in India, which include cardiovascular disease, arthritis, rheumatism, asthma, allergies, cancer, wound healing, metabolic and digestive problems, ulcers, eczema, viral diseases, especially hepatitis A and B, TB and senility.

What happens
In their traditional cultural role, non-medically qualified practitioners are known as *hakims*, and, because prevention is as important as cure, they advise on every aspect of the patient's life, including the choice of spouse. An initial consultation will include intensive questioning about everything from eating habits to relationships at work, and any remedies take into account the individual's constitution, astrological chart, age, mood, diet, the season, time of day and the climate – anything, in fact, that could possibly affect one's health and well-being. The practitioner also assesses build and facial features and pulse-taking is an important

part of the consultation. One reason Indian curries are so incredibly complicated to make is because of the requirement to balance energies in the food: for example, water-generating coriander must offset heat-inducing chilli.

Treatments prescribed include medicinal remedies prepared from herbs, minerals and vegetables; dietary advice; and practical therapies such as massage, steam baths and yoga.

Doctors say

Although records of Ayurvedic herbal preparations and their effects on humans go back centuries, there is no guarantee of the quality and efficacy of the remedies. As no thorough scientific analyses have been made of these mixtures, nobody knows which are the active ingredients, or whether they are effective on their own or only in combination with other substances.

Western doctors are happier with the *principles* of Ayurveda than many of its remedies, and anyone suffering from an acute condition such as appendicitis would be well advised to turn to orthodox medicine.

Rating

Popularity	Medical Credibility	Scientific Research	Availability
☆☆☆	☆☆☆	☆☆☆	☆☆

BACH FLOWER REMEDIES

Dr Edward Bach, a bacteriologist, physician and homeopath practising in London at the beginning of the century, believed that flowers could affect our state of mind and restore the balance necessary for good health. He identified 38 remedies by holding his hand over a plant, in the belief that he could intuitively recognise its healing properties. At first, only the dew on flowers was 'impregnated' with their healing qualities; later – dew being difficult to bottle in quantity – he decided that spring water would do as well, but only after the flower heads had floated in it, in full sunlight, for three hours.

Best for

Each remedy is associated with a different mood, emotion or personality type, rather than a specific complaint. Take gorse, for example, for feelings of hopelessness, or larch if you lack self-confidence. The 'Rescue Remedy', a composite of five remedies, is recommended for emergencies, to calm oneself after a sudden shock.

What happens

Dr Bach designed the remedies for self-help, but a number of practitioners in other fields – herbal medicine, homeopathy, naturopathy or those working with other flower and gem essences (see *Flower and gem essences*) – will prescribe Bach remedies in their treatment. The remedies are available from most health shops; they come in concentrated form and should be diluted with spring water.

Doctors say

Analysis shows that the remedies contain only spring water and alcohol, so any effects may be due to a molecular 'imprinting' similar to that claimed for homeopathy. Alternatively, the placebo effect of mind over body is very powerful: if you believe something will do you good, it often does.

Rating

Popularity	Medical Credibility	Scientific Research	Availability
✩✩✩	✩✩	✩	✩✩✩

THE BATES METHOD

This is a system of exercises to improve eyesight. Dr William Bates was a New York opthalmologist in the early twentieth century, who studied the way that our eyes change according to our physical and emotional state. He believed that many defects in vision are due to tension and poor function in the eye muscles and optic nerves, and devised a series of exercises that would relax and retrain the muscles.

The writer Aldous Huxley was one of Bates's great success stories. At age 45, Huxley was losing his eyesight, and turned to the Method. In two months, he reported, he could read without spectacles.

Best for

Those suffering from any conditions where glasses and contact lenses are prescribed, such as short and long sight, astigmatism and squint. For medical disorders such as glaucoma or cataracts, you should consult an orthodox eye specialist.

What happens

A Bates Method teacher will show you the basic exercises, and after that it is up to you. These exercises include:

Palming. This is claimed to enhance sight by resting the optic nerve and eye muscles. Remove spectacles or contact lenses and sit at a table with pillows supporting the elbows. Cover closed eyes with slightly cupped palms, fingers on the forehead, the idea being to shut out light without pressure on the eyes. Remain thus for at least ten minutes, two or three times a day, breathing deeply, relaxing and imagining deep blackness.

Swinging Swing rhythmically from side to side, eyes focused in the distance, but moving with your head.

Blinking Blink once or twice every ten seconds to clean and lubricate your eyes.

You will also receive advice on diet and nutritional supplements, and further exercises in memory and imagination to improve the feedback between eye and brain.

Doctors say

Eye exercises can improve sight in some cases, but these need a lot of dedication and perseverence. Do not expect miracles.

Rating

Popularity	Medical Credibility	Scientific Research	Availability
✭✭	✭✭	✭✭	✭✭

BIOCHEMIC TISSUE SALTS

Can everyday illnesses like colds and heartburn be due to a lack of essential inorganic minerals in the body? Biochemic tissue salts, such as fluoride of iron or chloride of soda, are recommended to restore the natural mineral balance.

'Tissue salts' and the study of 'biochemics' are terms coined by a German homeopathic physician, Dr Wilhelm Schuessler, in the 1870s. He claimed that many disorders could be blamed on a deficiency of one or more of twelve basic tissue salts. Later research supports some of his theories; people lacking enough calcium, for instance, are susceptible to nutrition and bone complaints.

The salts are homeopathic preparations, which means they are highly diluted. One part of the salt is mixed with nine parts of lactose (milk sugar) and this process is repeated another six times. They are taken as small tablets, dissolved on the tongue.

Best for

Minor ailments with recognisable symptoms, such as colds, coughs, indigestion, heartburn, cramp, neuralgia, muscular pain, minor skin conditions, headaches, sore throats, insomnia, catarrh, hay fever, cuts and burns.

What happens

Homeopaths, naturopaths and herbalists will often suggest tissue salts as part of a nutritional programme, but it is easy to dose yourself. Most health shops and some chemists stock tissue salts, and manufacturers usually provide accompanying information. Phosphate of iron (Ferr. Phos.), for example, is recommended for inflammations, minor injuries, early cold symptoms, sore throats, bronchitis and rheumatism.

Doctors say
The amount of active ingredient in the remedy is so small that it is harmless. Those with lactose intolerance could find the milk sugar base of the tablets upsetting. Otherwise, the only risk with self-dosing is that someone with a serious condition could put off seeking medical advice.

Rating

Popularity	Medical Credibility	Scientific Research	Availability
✮✮✮	✮✮	✮✮	✮✮✮

BIOENERGETICS

Practitioners believe that the life energy (akin to Qi and prana) which flows through our minds and bodies can become 'stuck'. Release often requires dramatic expression, both physically and emotionally.

Bioenergetics was a term first coined by Wilhelm Reich, a follower of Freud, who argued that an inability to achieve orgasm, and so release sexual energy through letting go of inhibitions, was the cause of many of our problems. He called this energy 'orgone', but in later life his experiments grew bizarre, and brought him to the attention of the United States police.

However, one of his students, Dr Alexander Lowen, retrieved the situation and developed a theory that our life stresses and traumas are programmed into our muscles, which become tense and painful. This state, known as 'body armouring', affects our breathing and body posture; arrogance and defiance, for example, may be reflected in a puffed chest and set jaw.

There are various schools of bioenergetics. One, known as biodynamics, was devised by Gerda Boyesen, who believed that we have an 'emotionally reactive' digestive system, and used massage to relieve stress. As a gauge to progress, the more the stomach rumbled, the more successful the therapy.

Best for
Stress-related conditions, such as irritable bowel syndrome, peptic ulcers, migraine, asthma, and anybody interested in personal growth, who wants to find out more about how they function in body and mind.

What happens
The initial assessment session is usually one-to-one. Later you may join a group of about eight or ten people for workshops and weekly meetings. There are various exercises and so-called 'stress positions' to 'unlock' energy, one of which involves lying backwards over a stool to build up an energy charge. Long-repressed memories of traumatic events from infancy may surface, and release often brings an outpouring of emotion; tears, anger and grief.

Doctors say
Very little. So far there is no scientific evidence of life energy, let alone any way of measuring it.

Rating

Popularity	Medical Credibility	Scientific Research	Availability
☆☆	☆☆	☆☆☆	☆☆

BIOFEEDBACK

People suffering from high blood pressure can lower it by consciously altering their brainwave pattern; others have eased migraine headaches by imagining their hands are cooler and lowering the electrical resistance of their skin. It is possible to learn to control a physical and mental condition through biofeedback, using equipment that measures changes in the body in a way that you can see or hear and respond to.

Blood pressure can be recorded, muscle tension can be registered on an electromyograph, and changes in brain wave patterns can be shown on an electroencephalograph. Nervous tension increases perspiration (the renowned 'sweaty palm' syndrome), so when electrodes attached to the palms of our hands are connected to a monitoring device, tiny changes in sweat production translate to figures on a screen. This is the science behind the success of the lie-detector.

Biofeedback began to be taken seriously when scientists researching brainwaves found that students could teach themselves to shift from one brainwave frequency to another at will. In everyday waking life, we are on the beta frequency. Alpha is a state of relaxed awareness, theta of drowsy day-dreaming, and delta is the frequency of deep sleep. When practitioners of transcendental meditation slipped into alpha, as Professor Herbert Benson of Harvard University discovered through biofeedback, their blood pressure was lowered.

Later studies showed that not only could people learn to raise or lower the temperature of their fingertips by using *autogenic training*, imagining their fingers as warmer or colder, but they did so more quickly if they could monitor their progress.

Best for
Stress-related conditions, such as high blood pressure, hyperventilation, insomnia, anxiety, tension headaches, migraine and some other kinds of muscle and joint pain.

What happens

The idea is to learn to recognise the mental and emotional states that accompany corresponding physiological responses so that they can be reproduced whenever required.

Electrodes are attached to the head (to measure brainwave frequencies), to the hands, or the part of the body whose responses are being measured. These electrodes are linked to the measuring device. Feedback is provided either by sound, a tone that varies with the measurement, or visually, with the movement of a needle, or colour changes. In Relaxplus, a sophisticated mind-controlled computer programme, developed at St Bartholomew's Hospital, the screen image of a mermaid changes into an angel as you relax.

Doctors say

Biofeedback demonstrably works, as literally thousands of scientific studies support, and numerous patients have weaned themselves off high-blood-pressure medication as a result. But how the mind overrules the involuntary workings of the autonomic nervous system is a mystery that is rapidly being unravelled through research into psychoneuroimmunology – the science of the mind–brain–body connection.

Rating

Popularity	Medical Credibility	Scientific Research	Availability
☆☆☆	☆☆☆	☆☆☆☆	☆☆☆

BIORHYTHMS

Although not stictly a therapy or self-help measure, a knowledge of your biorythms could help you plan your life for those times when you can perform at your optimum performance levels. There are days when nothing goes right, we have no energy, we cannot concentrate, and we snap at everyone. These could be 'critical periods' on our biorhythm chart, when internal 'clocks' that are said to govern our physical, emotional and intellectual capacities converge.

Biorhythms are calculated from the date of birth, and fall in three cycles: a 23-day *physical cycle* that is claimed to influence immunity, stamina, sex drive, confidence and accident-proneness; a 28-day *emotional cycle* influencing moods and creativity; and a 33-day *intellectual cycle* that affects decision-making, memory and concentration.

When charted, each cycle forms a wave pattern, moving between high, when energy peaks, to a passive low. Midpoints in the wave are said to be 'unstable' or 'critical' times, when anything can happen, especially if these periods occur on the same day for two or three cycles.

Biorhythms were first developed by a friend of Freud, Dr Wilhelm Fliess, who studied women's menstrual cycles. A contemporary Austrian psychologist, Professor Herman Swoboda, took the theory further, but it fell to an engineer, Professor Alfred Teltscher, to discover the intellectual cycle.

Best for
Planning holidays, surgical operations, business ventures, and any projects that depend on your top performance, or that involve risk. Some airline pilots take them very seriously.

Doctors say
The discovery of circadian (or daily) rhythms whetted scientific appetite for biorhythms. Concentration, for example, peaks measurably before you go to sleep, and sags in the after-lunch dip. Half of all heart attacks occur between 8 and 10 a.m. and 8 and 10 p.m. More people die in the early hours, and more babies are born at night.

Research has been ambivalent. An American psychologist, Professor Harold Willis, studied the records of patients who died in his local hospital in 1973, and found that over half of them expired on days that were individually critical for them. The same pattern also applied to the following year.

On the other hand, when the British Transport and Road Research

Laboratory compared the biorhythms of bus drivers in road accidents, there were no significant correlations. Other experts speculate that the situation may be complicated by the way different personalities react to stress. Being under pressure can put some people on their mettle.

Rating

Popularity	Medical Credibility	Scientific Research	Availability
✰✰✰	✰✰	✰✰✰	✰✰

CHIROPRACTIC

The term chiropractic comes from the Greek, 'cheiro' meaning hand, and 'praktikos', practice. A chiropractor uses the hands to manipulate joints and muscles – in particular those of the spine – to restore normal function to stiff joints and tight muscles.

When the vertebrae of the spine are even slightly stiff and dysfunctional, or under strain, not only can surrounding muscles, nerves and ligaments be affected, but problems can pop up almost anywhere because the spine protects a large part of the nervous system, which is the main 'telephone line' between the brain and every part of the body. A pinched nerve at the first cervical vertebra in the neck, for example, could be the cause of persistent migraine.

People often confuse chiropractic and osteopathy, as both treatments involve manipulation of the body. There are differences in the techniques they use but also, chiropractors tend to make more use of X-rays to look for the abnormal positions of the spine.

Chiropractic was developed by a Canadian osteopath, David Daniel (D.D.) Palmer. In 1895 he persuaded his office janitor, who had been deaf for 17 years after injuring his back and neck, to let him manipulate his spine. There was a 'click' and the man's hearing was restored.

Since then, chiropractic's reputation has fluctuated. After a dismal beginning when it was debunked as quackery, it soared in the early twentieth century, and plummeted again in the 1960s, when the American Medical Association condemned it as an 'unscientific cult'. Unable to prove this condemnation, the AMA lost a 12-year legal battle in 1987 and chiropractors are now allowed to practise in American hospitals.

In the UK, the word of satisfied patients was not enough, it seemed (93 per cent are happy customers), and, as a result, the chiropractic profession has worked assiduously on a dossier of positive research that would support its claim to be taken seriously.

One of the decisive studies was reported in the *British Medical Journal* in 1990. A Medical Research Council team found that patients receiving chiropractic treatment improved by 70 per cent more than those given normal hospital out-patient care.

In 1993, the King's Fund report into chiropractic called for the statutory regulation of practitioners, which would place them on a par with health professionals such as nurses and physiotherapists, and prevent unqualified 'rogue' practitioners setting themselves up as 'chiropractors'.

Now that the 1993 Osteopathy Act has given osteopaths legal status, chiropractic is expected to follow shortly.

Best for
Anything related to the spine and neck (sciatica, slipped discs, arm and shoulder pain and tension, lower back and lumbar pain, and sports injuries); rheumatism; gastrointestinal problems, such as indigestion and constipation; painful periods; postural problems associated with pregnancy and age; stress-related conditions; migraine; headaches; asthma; tinnitus and vertigo.

What happens
Although, like osteopathy, a 'biomechanical' treatment (i.e. manipulating bones and muscles), chiropractic also takes a holistic approach, regarding all aspects of life as influencing physical condition. A chiropractor begins with a detailed medical history, asks questions about lifestyle and notes posture and walking.

Chriopractor, Matthew Bennett, states:

> *'We will take into consideration diet, posture, how you sit at*
> *your desk at work, and even the patient's bed if we think these*
> *things are contributing to the problem.'*

In order to be physically examined, you will be expected to undress
to your underwear, although women are given a gown.

The chiropractor will probably do various tests: raising the legs,
moving the body from side to side, testing reflexes, and feeling the
effects of this on the spinal column.

Chiropractors take great care to ensure their diagnoses and
treatment are correct, backing up their observations with X-rays and
other standard medical tests, so that any other possible causes of
your condition are ruled out. If these do exist, you will be referred to
your GP, and, in any case, the practitioner will want to let your
doctor know that you are seeing a chiropractor.

Treatment proper usually begins at the second visit, when any
diagnostic tests have been returned. You stand, sit or lie on a
chiropractic couch; someone with severe back pain, for example,
can be lowered from a standing position on to a specially designed
couch. The chiropractor first moves the relevant spinal joint as far
as it will go (mobilisation), and then, with a rapid well-practised
thrust on the vertebra, takes it even further (manipulation). This
sudden stretching pulls and relaxes the muscles that are in spasm.

Because you have not had time to tense up and resist, this
'unlocking' of a joint is usually not painful, and often feels
immediately better. Some people may feel a little stiff and achy later,
but it wears off. Depending on the severity of the problem, you may
have to return for a number of treatments.

An initial session can last 45 to 60 minutes, although subsequent
ones tend to be shorter. Average fees for a first visit are £35 to £40,
more if X-rays are taken, and later ones about £18.

David, a 43-year-old signwriter and mural artist went to a
chiropractor:

> *'Injuries from playing football in my youth had weakened my*
> *back. Last summer, as I was working, bending up and down to*

apply lettering, my back suddenly wrenched and I couldn't move for two days. I couldn't even lift a tea cup. I'd been in pain for about a week when I saw an ad in the paper for National Back Pain Week and the freephone number for a local chiropractor.

'Not only did he say he could help, but he said it was straightforward, which surprised me, as I'd thought the weakness was permanent. He told me I would need about eight treatments, and I went back a week later for the first one. It didn't take long, about 15 minutes. He said I had an extremely stiff neck, and did some manipulations. Afterwards, I found myself lifting calor gas bottles without thinking about it.*

'I've been seven times now, once a week for the first four and then fortnightly, and I've felt slight improvements after each session. I sit on the table, and he moves my neck from side to side; then I lie down in the recovery position, he puts wedges under me and pushes hard on my back, and the joints seem to 'click'. It took my breath away the first time, but it's not painful.*

'Last week was a good test – I was bending up and down all day, and fell into bed physically exhausted, but I had no aches or pains that night or the next day, as I would normally expect. I still feel there's a slight weakness, but the improvement has been wonderful. Already I feel better than I can remember in years.*

'The chiropractor told me the problem was not in my back or neck, but at t*h*e top of the groin on the left hand side, probably an old football injury even though I'd never had pain there.'*

Doctors say

Chiropractic is now taken seriously by the medical profession, and should soon be part of the NHS. Many doctors will refer patients to a chiropractor for musculo-skeletal problems.

Rating

Popularity	Medical Credibility	Scientific Research	Availability
✰✰✰✰	✰✰✰	✰✰✰✰	✰✰✰✰

McTimoney and McTimoney-Corley chiropractic

These are simpler and gentler forms of chiropractic, developed by John McTimoney and Hugh Corley, applied to joints all over the body where bones have lost their alignment. Specially trained practitioners work with animals, with the approval of a veterinary surgeon.

Training is comparatively short at present, although the four-year, part-time study course at the McTimoney Chiropractic School and Witney School of Chiropractic will be upgraded to comply with future regulations. McTimoney chiropractors use the letters MC (McTimoney Chiropractor) and belong to the McTimoney Chiropractic Association (MCA). Graduates of the Witney School belong to the British Association of Applied Chiropractic.

CLINICAL ECOLOGY

Clinical ecologists treat disorders which, they believe, result from our reactions to the environment in which we live. This is known as environmental medicine.

Allergies to certain foods and substances – wheat and dairy products, for example – have been around for years. Now there is growing suspicion that many more people are becoming sensitive to chemicals in the environment, such as petrol fumes, weedkillers and household cleaners, and in food preparation and preservation. Our bodies cope with this onslaught of stress and pollution for a while, and then collapse in one way or another. Convalescence after a viral infection such as 'flu, when the immune system has taken a pounding, can be an especially vulnerable time.

Best for
The environment has been blamed for asthma, headaches, stomach upsets, fatigue, rheumatoid arthritis, psoriasis, eczema, bloating, water retention, rapid weight fluctuations, dizziness and depression.

What happens
The clinical ecologist will examine you to check general health and

ask questions about your medical history and lifestyle for evidence of exposure to various substances. Then one or all of the following tests will be suggested. The first two involve taking a blood sample.

Leucocytotoxic test Checks the reaction of white blood cells to food extracts.

Blood test Measures the components of the blood to detect mineral levels and immune function.

Vega test When a substance is placed on the machine, electrodes on your acupuncture points record your response.

Applied kinesiology Checks if substances on your tongue or in your hand cause muscle weakening. (see *Kinesiology*)

Auriculo-cardiac reflex method Suspect substances are said to speed up your pulse when placed on your skin.

Hair analysis Identifies high levels of toxic metals or low levels of minerals.

The simplest methods of diagnosis and treatment may include elimination or rotation diets (you begin by eating a few foods, and gradually add more until one provokes a reaction), avoiding the substances you are allergic to, and nutritional supplements (see *Nutritional therapy*). A more exotic (and expensive) treatment is enzyme potentiated desensitisation: to suppress your reaction, the suspect substance is mixed with an enzyme and injected or applied to your skin.

Clinical ecology is not available on the NHS, so it is wise to check how much a course of treatment will cost beforehand: an initial consultation can cost £30 to £100.

Doctors say

Orthodox opinion is divided about this controversial therapy, especially about the methods of diagnosis and treatment. Even some clinical ecologists are wary of the more fringe treatments, such as the vega test or auriculo-cardiac reflex method. Research has shown that some treatments are no better than a placebo, but a number of patients have claimed almost miraculous relief.

Rating

Popularity	Medical Credibility	Scientific Research	Availability
✫✫✫	✫✫✫	✫✫✫	✫✫✫

COLONIC IRRIGATION

This currently popular therapy, also known as colonic hydrotherapy, is said to be favoured by less conventional members of the Royal Family. According to practitioners, years of over-processed food and mucus-inducing dairy products have resulted in 'auto-intoxication' or self-poisoning. The bowel and large intestine are clogged with impacted waste matter, they claim, and populated with micro-organisms that do not help us feel well. This is the cause of most health problems, from acne and eczema to fibroids and constipation. Toxins have nowhere to go but back into our body systems, so the solution is to flush everything out. Literally.

What happens

A tube is inserted into the rectum, and warm water flows, under gentle gravitational pressure, into the large intestine via a small tube, softening the waste material and cleansing the bowel of years of accumulated debris. This is then carried away in a transparent evacuation tube.

Emma, a 31-year-old secretary, described her 'awesome' experience:

> *'I'd imagined a huge rush of water, but I didn't feel anything. It wasn't at all degrading or embarrassing, though I didn't particularly like the sensation. But the next day I felt great, cleaner and lighter. I'd lost two pounds in weight.'*

Colonic practitioners recommend a change of diet and an initial series of four to eight colonics. Healthy bowel bacteria are encouraged with capsules of *Lactobacillus acidophilus* and a herbal tonic. A healthy bowel, they say, will evacuate two or three times a day after meals.

Doctors say

Medical opinion ranges from cautious to scathing. One gastroenterologist felt that a single treatment might be of some help in chronic constipation, a medically underestimated problem in women, and difficult to treat. But gastroenterologist, Dr Parveen Kumar, of St Bartholomew's Hospital, London, stated:

> *This is potentially dangerous and of no proven benefit. The bowel contains a lot of antigens and bacteria, but these cause no harmful effects, and all faecal matter is passed out of the body throught the rectum. Water absorption from the large volume of fluid irrigated could cause heart failure in some people.*

About claims to feel better and lighter, she said: 'A placebo effect.' Mucus and impacted debris? 'The water can irritate the colonic mucosa and produce mucus. It is not harmful, and most people don't have impacted debris.' Defaecation thrice daily? 'A healthy person defaecates anything from three times a day to once every three to four days. It is not necessary to go daily.'

Rating

Popularity	Medical Credibility	Scientific Research	Availability
✮✮	✮	✮✮	✮✮

COLOUR THERAPY

American psychologists discovered that prisoners calmed down and became more amenable when cell walls were painted a particular shade of pink, said to be the same as the inside of the womb. Certainly colour has an undeniable impact on us. We talk of 'feeling blue', 'seeing red', going 'green' with jealousy. Interior decorators and paint manufacturers as well as psychologists know that colour affects mood and concentration: blue is soothing in bedrooms, red can make a dull lecture seem exciting and stimulates appetite (Indian restaurants use red flock wallpaper to good effect!). We have individual colour preferences: one person finds a particular shade of blue restful, another finds it depressing. A green sweater in which you feel vibrant could leave your friend feeling washed out and queasy.

The electromagnetic wavelengths of light from the sun include those that are visible as colours of the spectrum – red, yellow, orange, green, blue, indigo, violet – and those that are invisible to the human eye, such as ultraviolet and infrared, both of which are known to have healing properties.

Colour therapists believe that the body absorbs these various electromagnetic wavelengths of light and emits an aura of its own, the colours of which will reflect your current physical, emotional and spiritual health.

Best for
Practitioners claim that almost any condition can be treated, especially depression, ME (myalgic encephalomyelitis), stress-related problems, and learning difficulties.

What happens
At the first consultation, you will be asked to fill out a form with details of your medical history and your preferences for particular colours. The practitioner places this under a spine chart, where each vertebra is associated with a colour, and uses a finger to 'dowse' the colours needed for treatment. This could mean sitting in coloured light for a certain period, or visualising and surrounding yourself with therapeutic colours. Other practitioners work with the *chakras*, or energy centres of the body, each of which is associated with a different colour and corresponding emotion.

Sessions are usually monthly, for nine to twelve months, at about £25 per session.

Doctors say
There is plenty of evidence that colour affects our mood and behaviour. American psychologist, Dr Max Luscher, devised a personality test based on colour preferences that has been used for job selection. In a Norwegian study, people in a blue room set the thermomostat three degrees higher than those in a red room. But while there is no harm in making the most of a favourite shade,

when it comes to auras and dowsing most orthodox practitioners remain sceptical.

Rating

Popularity	Medical Credibility	Scientific Research	Availability
☆	☆☆	☆☆	☆☆

CRANIAL OSTEOPATHY (see OSTEOPATHY)

Many osteopaths have undergone training in cranial osteopathic techniques. The bones that make up our skull (or cranium) are not fixed but can move very slightly, a flexibility necessary at birth, when the baby's head has to negotiate the birth canal. If these bones and other body tissues do not ease correctly back into place, however, or are knocked even marginally out of position later in life, osteopaths who use cranial techniques believe that subtle body movements, known as the cranial rhythmic impulse (CRI), may be disturbed, causing symptoms of dysfunction throughout the body.

By very gentle and delicate manipulation, cradling the body and working with the CRI, practitioners coax the tissues back into a more normal working relationship, thus restoring health and ease.

Andrew Taylor Still, an American doctor, founded osteopathy in the 1870s. The 'Cranial' approach was a further development of Still's ideas at the turn of the century by William Garner Sutherland, an osteopath trained by Still.

Best for

Major and minor strains and sprains where other treatment has failed, especially resulting from road traffic accidents or falls, pregnancy and delivery; head and spinal injuries, face, mouth and jaw pain, sinusitis; arthritic problems; irritable bowel and constipation; menstrual discomfort; post-operative pain, often resulting from scar tissue or adhesions; recurrent infections,

particularly in children; newborn babies whose heads have
been distorted by a difficult birth.

What happens

You should ensure that you see an osteopath who is also fully
trained in cranial osteopathic techniques. The practitioner will take
your medical history and ask you about your lifestyle and general
health, before deciding whether cranial osteopathic treatment is
appropriate for your condition, or whether another form of
osteopathy would be more suitable.

You will probably have to undress down to your underwear before
lying on a special treatment couch, as the osteopath works on the
shoulders, spine and pelvis, as well as the head, to restore normal
tissue movement and balance.

The manipulation is very gentle and so subtle that it may feel as if
hardly anything is happening. Several sessions may be required to sort
out the problem; these cost about £20 to £30 each and are not widely
available on the NHS. While a doctor's reference is not necessary, the
osteopath will wish to inform your GP, with your consent.

Doctors say

Cranial osteopathy is still regarded with suspicion by some doctors,
and even some osteopaths hold it to be on the perimeter of
osteopathic therapy. However, in trained hands, remarkable results
seem possible.

Rating

Popularity	Medical Credibility	Scientific Research	Availability
✫✫✫	✫✫✫	✫✫	✫✫✫

CRANIO-SACRAL THERAPY

The basic approach and some of the manipulative techniques of this
therapy are similar to *Cranial Osteopathy*, though without the ground-

ing in osteopathy. Cranio-sacral practitioners favour the theories of a controversial American osteopath, Dr John Upledger, who claims that the cranial rhythm pulses throughout the whole body.

The cranio-sacral system is described as the bones of the cranium and sacrum; the membranes surrounding the brain and spinal cord, enclosing the cerebro-spinal fluid; and the fascia, the fibrous tissue connecting the muscles.

It is believed that strains in the symmetrical rhythm of the cerebro-spinal fluid can cause physical and emotional disorders. Practitioners gently pull and twist the connective tissue all over the body until they feel symmetry is restored.

Best for

Cranio-sacral therapy claims to treat the whole person, and therefore will benefit almost any condition. Specialities include headache, asthma, arthritis, digestive problems, spinal curvatures, anxiety, fatigue, post-viral syndrome, after effects of meningitis and head injury.

Doctors say

Anyone cautious of cranial osteopathy will be even more sceptical of this. There is real concern among osteopaths that cranio-sacral practitioners, however well-meaning, lack adequate clinical training. In itself, the massage is harmless and soothing, but as people tend to seek such practitioners because of a specific problem, a serious medical condition could be overlooked or given dangerously wrong treatment.

Rating

Popularity	Medical Credibility	Scientific Research	Availability
☆☆☆	☆☆	☆☆	☆☆☆

CRYSTAL AND GEM HEALING

A belief that crystal rocks and precious and semi-precious gems have special mystic and therapeutic qualities is found in traditions, both ancient and modern, around the world. Different stones are said to resonate at varying vibrational levels of energy, and thus have particular qualities that can interact with one's own healing and creative energy. Quartz, for example, is used for general healing; garnet is said to protect against depression and skin diseases; malachite helps asthma, toothache and irregular periods.

Much is claimed for the power of crystals, and there are currently any number of books and consultants that provide information, and shops that sell crystals. One or more crystals may be kept as personal sources of healing and tended with care. They are said to like to lie on silk or black velvet.

What happens

It is a good idea to ask what will happen, as healers' techniques vary. After some questions about your lifestyle and medical history, you may sit in a chair, or lie on a couch, a futon or the floor, while the healer arranges crystals around you, or puts stones on your body. Unless the treatment is combined with aromatherapy (practitioners are often trained in other therapies), you will not be asked to undress. Sessions last 30 to 90 minutes, and fees range from a donation to about £35.

Doctors say

There is no scientific evidence that crystals possess healing powers. But if you believe they can help you, there is no harm in using them – so long as you also consult an orthodox medical practitioner with any symptoms of ill health.

Rating

Popularity	Medical Credibility	Scientific Research	Availability
✭✭✭	✭	✭	✭✭

DANCE MOVEMENT THERAPY

The power of dance to take you out of yourself is very ancient. Dance therapy as such made its appearance in the US in the 1940s, but did not get off the ground in the UK until much later. Although first used to help those with mental health problems, 'healthy' people discovered that dance, unchoreographed and instinctive, enabled them to get in touch with inner feelings too deep for words, and express them as movements.

Best for
It will help the average person to unwind and keep fit; those with depression and anxiety; institutionalised mental patients; the blind and physically disabled; post-operative patients; children and young people with autism, learning difficulties and behavioural problems.

What happens
Almost anything may happen, as dance therapists have very individual approaches. A session usually begins with loosening up exercises. Circle dancing is immensely popular in personal growth workshops. 'Holding hands and moving round together, stamping our feet, was tremendously liberating,' said a 45-year-old college lecturer. 'You had the same sense of fun and group support as in childhood.'

Music is not always necessary. Rhythm can be made with feet, hands, legs. Sometimes practitioners encourage exercises such as 'rolling over bridges', where you explore climbing over a partner's back.

Doctors say
There is no doubt about the benefits of dance therapy for those with physical disabilities, the mentally ill and those with emotional disorders. Others usually find it very enjoyable, regardless of age, skill, or fitness – though sufferers from back pain or high blood pressure would be advised to check with a doctor before doing vigorous exercise.

Rating

Popularity	Medical Credibility	Scientific Research	Availability
★★	★★	★★	★★

DO-IN

This has been described as a self-help version of *acupressure* and *shiatsu*. Pronounced 'dough-in', it is a home health maintenance programme, traditionally popular in China and Japan, consisting of a series of simple stretching and breathing exercises that massage the meridians or energy channels of the body.

Rating

Popularity	Medical Credibility	Scientific Research	Availability
★	★★	★	★

DOWSING

It is a little disconcerting when a practitioner pulls out a pendulum on the end of a silk thread and holds it over your abdomen, letting it swing back and forth before announcing that your gall bladder is in need of repair. Dowsing appears in a number of therapies – aromatherapists, herbalists and homeopaths sometimes use it to confirm decisions – although as a diagnostic tool it is most closely aligned with radionics.

Traditionally, dowsers located subterranean water with a hazelwood divining rod. Learning that some also claimed to know if an underground stream was 'evil' and would affect the health of those living about it, Abbé Mermet, a French priest, applied the technique in the 1920s, to patients in the local hospital, with some success.

According to his theory, which became the basis for radionics, all substances in the body emit 'good' and 'bad' vibrations, rather like radio sound waves, which can be picked up by a sensitive dowser. Later researchers found that the technique could be used on parts of the whole body – hair, blood, urine and so on. A clockwise swing usually means 'yes', anti-clockwise 'no'.

Doctors say
Very little.

Rating

Popularity	Medical Credibility	Scientific Research	Availability
☆☆	☆	☆	☆☆

THE FELDENKRAIS METHOD

Moshe Feldenkrais was a Russian-born Israeli physicist and engineer who escaped through France during World War II and settled in the UK. Because he was a judo teacher and keen soccer player, a knee injury left him more determined than most to walk again without pain. A combination of science and martial arts, plus a study of yoga, the Alexander Technique and the spontaneous, natural grace of children, led to the development of his Method, aimed at developing ease of movement with what he called 'minimum effort and maximum efficiency'.

Students of the Method learn to be constantly aware of their body, so they can recognise muscle tension and respond by reorganising their movements. This improves posture and circulation and creates a sense of well-being. For example, someone suffering from depression often stoops and has hunched shoulders. When taught to change their pattern of movement, they straighten up and (so the theory goes) stop being depressed.

Best for

General fitness, chronic pain, injury trauma, back pain, strokes, paralysis, scoliosis, cerebral palsy and learning disabilities. Actors, dancers and athletes benefit too.

What happens

Students learn the Method either in groups, known as 'awareness through movement', or individually, called 'functional integration'. The latter is more practical than theoretical, and especially useful for people with disabilities.

To begin with, exercises are taught while the student is lying on the floor, to reduce the effects of gravity on the joints. Breathing is an important part of the gentle, relaxed movements.

Doctors say

Like the Alexander Technique, anything that improves posture, breathing and muscular function – especially in the disabled and elderly – is likely to be beneficial.

Rating

Popularity	Medical Credibility	Scientific Research	Availability
☆☆	☆☆☆	☆☆	☆☆

FLOATATION THERAPY

You climb into what, from the outside, appears to be a home sauna. Inside is a large bath about 8 feet by 4 feet, with water 10 inches deep, and so packed with Epsom salts that you float effortlessly, as if you were in the Dead Sea. The temperature of this solution is maintained at 34.2 degrees Centrigade, the same as that of the skin, so that there is no sensation of being in water, no external sensations at all. The door is closed, the light switched off, and earplugs keep out external noise. You remain there for the next 45, 60 or 150 minutes.

Relatively easily and quickly, this treatment induces an extremely deep state of mental and physical relaxation. Stressed individuals, who have difficulty relaxing by other means, often find that floatation enables them to wind down. Most tanks also have speakers, and you can listen to *hypnotherapy* or *meditation* tapes to encourage you to give up smoking, become more self-confident, or whatever.

Best for
Stress-related conditions, such as high blood pressure, ulcers, migraine, headaches, cardiovascular disease, anxiety, immune system suppression; back pain; muscle fatigue; pain control; addiction.

What happens
You are given a towel and earplugs and shown the float tank or pool in a private room with a shower, which you use before and after entering the water. Most people float naked. Claustrophobics need not be anxious: a light in the tank can be switched on and off whenever you wish, and the door opened from inside at any time. Water should be filtered and recycled after each float session, although the high concentration of salts wipes out viruses and bacteria.

Tom, a 38-year-old manager gave his impression:

> *'Rather creepy to begin with, and I wondered how I was going to stand an hour of it, but after a while your mind calms down and wanders into all kinds of avenues, and the next thing you know the dolphin music they play to signal the end of the float has come on. I felt refreshed afterwards, and rather spaced out for a while.'*

Doctors say
Floatation evolved from the studies of an American psychoanalyst and neuro-physiologist, Dr John C. Lilly, into the reactions of the brain when denied external stimulation. Further research has shown that it is effective in reducing stress biochemicals and affecting endocrinal and psychological states. Pain relief and a sense of mild euphoria is due to the release of endorphins, the body's natural painkillers.

Warning

Although severe anxiety, phobias and depression can be alleviated by floatation therapy, anyone suffering from these conditions should not use a tank without professional supervision.

Rating

Popularity	Medical Credibility	Scientific Research	Availability
✮✮✮	✮✮✮	✮✮	✮✮✮

FLOWER AND GEM ESSENCES

This is an extension of the *Bach flower remedies*. In the 1970s an American, Richard Katz, realised that the power of flower essences was not limited to 38 English plants. He began by bottling 70 Californian flower essences, said to contain vibrations of the sun's energy, absorbed by the petals of flowers when left in sun-warmed water. That was the start of a flood of flower essences from around the globe, notably the Himalayas and the Australian bush. Some companies now market gem essences too, allegedly trapping the energy of precious and semi-precious stones in a similar way.

Flower essences, it is believed, have a healing power that can re-establish the link between body and soul. When these are out of harmony, we are susceptible to disease; when connected, the sense of wholeness energises the body's self-healing powers.

What happens

With so many essences now available, it is difficult to find something appropriate without expert help. A consultation with Clare Harvey, who specialises in Bach Flower Remedies and flower and gem essences, begins with questions about your medical history and lifestyle. There are literally hundreds of bottles to choose from, so she uses a kind of dowsing method to find the right essence. You place your finger on a bottle, or group of bottles, and she places her finger on yours. Partly from intuition, she says, partly from sensing vibrations, she knows which to choose. A maximum of five essences are added to an alcohol base in a fresh bottle, from which you are told to take three drops in a couple of centimetres of water every morning.

Doctors say

Most doctors are very sceptical of the claims for the essences' healing powers, but, provided you consult your GP with any symptoms of illness, there is no harm in trying them.

Rating

Popularity	Medical Credibility	Scientific Research	Availability
✭✭	✭✭	✭	✭✭✭

HEALING

Healers describe what they do as restoring to health by non-physical means, either through the hands, or at a distance by thought or prayer, or by radionic instrument (see *Radionics*). Explanations vary according to the healer's beliefs and procedures, but it generally involves what the Confederation of Healing Organisations (CHO) calls 'a transference of harmonising paraphysical energies.'

The body, mind and soul are seen as a partnership, and well-being as homeostasis – the natural equilibrium between all parts of an entity. Illness is said to result from a disorder in this partnership.

A favourite analogy is that of a car (the body) and driver (mind and spirit). If the driver is drunk or lost, then the car, no matter how powerful or well-maintained, is going nowhere. Both car and driver are part of the package, as it were – except that it is the driver who makes the decisions. Our mind and spirit influences our health, and it's not uncommon to hear it said that a patient died because the 'will to live' was lost.

What a healer supposedly can do is channel the energies needed to regenerate our self-healing abilities, and put us back into the driving seat.

Where does this 'life energy' come from? Among spiritual healers, Christians would say God, someone from the Chinese tradition would talk of Qi, an Indian of *prana*. Those of no religious allegiance might ascribe it to the power of love, a 'cosmic force', or, with a sidelong glance at quantum physics, a dynamic energy that pulses through the universe. Spiritualist (not the same as spiritual) healers claim that a discarnate entity from the spirit world takes over while they are in a trance; George Chapman, for example, says he becomes a channel for Dr William Lang, an English eye surgeon who died in 1937 and who performs operations on the patient's 'spirit' body.

All these involve the idea of transmission of energy from some benign source, and do not necessarily depend on whether the patient believes in the healer or not. In fact, there are cases where animals, and even plants, have been helped by a healer.

There is another, generally frowned-on practice known as 'faith' healing, in which any improvement depends on the patient's faith and trust in either the personal powers of the healer or the person or cult leader he or she represents. No belief: no cure. As a rule, beware of anyone who makes extortionate demands in return for healing, whether of large sums of money, of belief, or of commitment. Almost by definition, healing is a power that is freely given; all we have to do is receive.

As with many other therapies, improvement is often said to occur more readily when the patient feels a rapport with the healer, and is responsive to the idea of healing. Strange as it may seem, some people are – consciously or unconsciously –resistant to getting better.

Tonie, a travel agent, was so impressed with her therapy that she eventually became a healer herself:

> *'My knee was damaged in a car accident. Chips of bone had lodged in my knee joint and it stiffened so that I couldn't bend it. I saw a physiotherapist for months, who finally said there was*

nothing she could do, and then I heard by chance of a healer. After a year of monthly visits, my knee gradually eased up until I could sit back on my heels. That was twenty years ago, and the only result of the accident now is that one leg is slightly longer than the other.'

Best for

All conditions that afflict the body, mind and spirit may be relieved, though not necessarily cured, by healing. Although there have been claims of miraculous cures, the throwing away of crutches and melting of tumours, in many instances the condition remains, but the patient's pain is alleviated or they *feel* better and their quality of life is improved.

What happens

Healers work by several methods. One, the simplest and oldest, is contact healing, often known as *laying on of hands*. It is a natural instinct: when someone is ill or upset, many of us intuitively touch them; a comforting arm around the shoulder perhaps, or a hand on the arm.

Contact healers use their hands as amplifiers and conduits of healing power, placing them on the site of the disease, or making a series of strokes or 'passes' a few centimetres above the body. Energy implies heat, and the healer's hands may indeed feel hot. Patients often report a warm, tingling sensation, and a feeling of calm and relaxation (see *Therapeutic Touch*).

Some healers might work with the *aura*, a field of radiance that they claim to see emanating from people. The colours in the aura are said to reflect a person's state of health, grey and muddy brown being particularly unwholesome (see *Colour therapy*). Such healers might place their hands on the aura and visualise vibrant colours such as green or orange.

You may consult a healer in a centre or clinic, at his or her home, or even in a GP's surgery. The atmosphere should be calm and peaceful (be wary of healers who seem irritable and in a rush), and there may be candles or soft music to enhance such an atmosphere. You will be asked questions about your complaint, general health, medical history and lifestyle. You should be asked if you have been to your doctor, and recommended to do so if you have not, especially if the healer is a member of one of the organisations belonging to the Confederation of Healers. The healer will probably then ask you to make yourself comfortable, either sitting or lying down on a couch, while they sit or stand alongside and attune themselves to you.

Brainwave researchers, such as Maxwell Cade, found that in the healing process, a healer's brainwave frequency slipped into alpha, a state of relaxed awareness also found in meditation (see *Biofeedback*) and was followed within seconds by that of the patient. Jean Roberton, a healer who is also a GP, asks that her patients attend several lessons in *meditation* to prepare for healing.

Once attuned, the healer concentrates on the patient, opens the mind to whatever source of healing energy they perceive, and allows this to flow through them into the patient. One healer, for instance, pictures a stream of pure white light that splits into rainbow colours.

> *'All the colours come up into my heart energy centre and then come out of my hands. Both my patients and I experience warmth when this happens.'*

In *absent* or *distant healing*, of which prayer is an obvious example, a healer or group of healers, often at a prearranged time, visualise healing energy transferring from themselves to the distant recipient.

Some people say they feel better immediately after healing, others report that it can take hours, days, or occasionally weeks or at least several visits before experiencing benefits – if any. Paradoxically, conditions which were not mentioned may clear up, while the original complaint remains unchanged.

Doctors say

Although conventional medical practitioners are generally sceptical and point out that scientific proof of a healing energy has yet to be definitively established, many are open-minded and even wholeheartedly supportive. There is enough anecdotal evidence to indicate that *something* is happening, even if it is a placebo effect or auto-suggestion (healing by self-hypnosis).

Provided the funding comes from the practice budget, and the doctor retains clinical responsibility, a GP may refer a patient to a healer on the NHS. Hospitals, hospices and pain clinics are making increasing use of healers – the CHO estimates that more than 200 registered healers worked in hospitals over the last year.

A number of scientific studies have shown the beneficial effects of healing. Recent research in the UK on people with arthritis and with leg ulcers indicates that, although their physical condition was unchanged, healing can make patients feel better and play a part in relieving suffering. The research teams wish to repeat the trials on a larger scale, but no finance has been available to date.

Dr Daniel Benor, an American psychiatrist and healer working in the UK, has researched the literature available, and claims there are numerous controlled studies demonstrating the positive effects of healing. Healers, including the British psychic Matthew Manning, have successfully increased wound healing in mice and humans, extended the life of blood cells, speeded the growth of plant cells and raised the activity of enzymes. However, because of its subjective nature, healing does not always take kindly to laboratory conditions, and there have been many failures too.

Rating

Popularity	Medical Credibility	Scientific Research	Availability
✫✫✫✫	✫✫✫	✫✫✫	✫✫✫✫

HERBALISM

Herbal is the adjective of the moment: herbal tea, herbal shampoo, herbal cosmetics... As one synthetic drug after another is discovered to have unwelcome, and sometimes lethal, side effects, a disenchanted public finds nature's own products increasingly attractive.

The picture is one of sun-drenched flower-strewn meadows, lavender by the door and bouquets of herbs above the rustic range in the cottage kitchen. Even a leading chain of chemists has joined in with its own brand of herbal remedies.

But herbal medicine is more than a soothing cup of camomile tea, or a hop pillow for insomnia. Anne McIntyre, one of Britain's leading medical herbalists, wrote in her book *Herbal Medicine*: 'Herbalism is a system of medicine in its own right, offering treatment for a wide variety of illnesses.'

'Herbs' are not just the handful of rosemary and sage leaves you might toss into the cooking pot, but any plant, including flowers or trees, that can benefit health.

The pharmaceutical industry has already raided the plant world for drugs. Digoxin is one example. When heart patients he expected to die astonished him by getting better, an eighteenth century English doctor, William Withering, found that an old village woman was dosing them with foxglove. The botanical name of this plant is digitalis, and digoxin, the therapeutic agent, is now a synthesised ingredient in modern heart disease drugs.

A herbalist would never isolate a plant substance in this way, believing that a remedy works because of the delicate chemical balance of the whole plant. When extracted and used on its own, the active agent can have side effects which are negated by other substances in the same plant.

The plant, meadowsweet, is the herbal equivalent of aspirin, because it contains salicylic acid which, in isolation, can cause internal bleeding in people with sensitive stomach linings. But meadowsweet also contains tannin and mucilage, natural protectors and healers of the stomach lining, and is actually used for a whole range of digestive disorders.

Rather than treating symptoms in isolation, herbal medicine seeks to restore what it calls 'the vital force', the body's own capacity to protect, regulate, renew and heal itself – physically, mentally and emotionally. Eczema is a manifestation of the body's attempt to restore balance, or 'homeostasis'; a herbalist will not just hand you a cream for the rash, but will try to find the source of the problem. Is it caused by poor diet, or an unhealthy lifestyle? Is the individual carrying an unusual burden of stress that is upsetting the delicate balance of the body? What natural remedy or change in diet will restore harmony and natural cleansing?

Animals instinctively know what herbs to eat if wounded or bitten, and our earliest use of herbal remedies was probably intuitive. Ancient Chinese and Egyptian records over two thousand years old refer to herbal medicine, and the great Greek doctors, Hippocrates and Galen, practised herbalism. In England, Nicolas Culpeper wrote a definitive book on herbs in 1649.

As chemical compounds began to be used in medicine, herbalism fell out of favour, relegated to folksy old women in the countryside. Although herbal medicine flourished in other countries, especially China, India and South America, its survival in the West was largely thanks to the Pilgrim Fathers in America. They added new Indian remedies to their own herblore, and herbal schools and societies were soon well established in the US. In 1864 an English doctor brought the American system of herbal medicine back to Britain, and the National Association of Medical Herbalists (now the Institute of Medical Herbalists) was established.

The discovery of penicillin and other wonder drugs in the twentieth century offered the distracting promise of magic cures for a number of years, but herbal remedies are now finding a place in healthcare. Even such arcane habits as gathering herbs by moonlight as the dew forms have been validated: science has shown that belladonna and the opium poppy contain higher concentrations of their medical properties in the early morning.

Best for

Most illnesses, including chronic (longstanding) conditions such as migraine, arthritis, cystitis, skin complaints, hormonal and digestive problems. For any condition requiring complicated tests or surgery (cancer, appendicitis) you would be referred immediately to a conventional doctor, or, for musculo-skeletal problems, to a chiropractor or osteopath.

What happens

On the first visit, which usually lasts at least an hour, the herbalist will take a detailed medical history, going right back to early childhood and even infancy. Were you breastfed and for how long?

You will be asked about your lifestyle, diet, mental and emotional state – including recent bereavements or marital problems. There may be a simple physical examination, even a gynaecological examination if necessary, and tests such as blood pressure and vision. Under the 1968 Medicines Act a qualified herbalist may prescribe medications, so it is important to obtain as much information as possible before making a diagnosis.

Usually any herbal remedy will be made up there and then, and you are asked to report back in a week or two, earlier if your condition is acute. Remedies may work in a few days, although chronic conditions usually take longer. Fees are usually about £28 for the first consultation and £18 for subsequent visits; more if you live around London.

Gail, aged 49, a married woman with two sons at university recounted her experience.

'I'd been having a few problems with the menopause. Hot flushes and depression. We'd had a lot of financial problems too and I felt suicidal. My doctor prescribed HRT and it worked reasonably well for a couple of months and then became a total disaster. My husband said I was liveable with for only ten days of the month. A local herbalist had given a talk to the WI, and I was desperate enough to try anything.

'I thought it would be like a visit to the doctor, a few tests, take this, but she was so sympathetic. We chatted for an hour and a half about my life and childhood, how I ate and slept, and then she put me on this horrendous medicine that tasted absolutely foul.

'You'll get used to it,' she said, and it was true. It was a mixture of herbs to help my nervous and hormonal systems cope on their own, and I took it three times a day after meals. I'd see her once a month, and we'd talk about all sorts of things as if we were friends; there was never any impression of a hurry. She suggested I take multivitamins and evening primrose oil as well, and advised me to give up caffeine and eat more hot food.

'In two or three weeks I had started to improve, and five months later she signed me off. Now I feel wonderful, and everyone says I look so much better.'

Self-help

Although the most potent prescriptions are those mixed by a medical herbalist, there are still a number of effective commercially produced creams, ointments, essential oils, tinctures and teas available in health shops and some chemists. Simple remedies can even be grown in your garden, and prepared as compress and poultice dressings for wounds, bruises and infections.

Herbal drinks come in various forms:

decoction Powdered or dried herbs are simmered for 20 minutes, strained, and the resulting tea drunk while hot.

tincture This is the most common form of remedy prescribed by herbalists. Herbs are steeped in alcohol or glycerol for two weeks, strained, and are then ready for use.

infusion This is the easiest way to make a herbal drink at home. Warm a teapot, and put in one dessertspoonful of herb per cup. Add a cup of boiling water for each cup required. Leave it to infuse for 10 to 15 minutes.

tisane The herbs are sold in the form of teabags, add boiling water and leave to brew for a minute or two.

Herbal first aid

Cuts Apply tincture of calendula (single marigold) and St John's wort, or (the commercial variation) Hypercal ointment. In an emergency, a marigold flower crushed on to the cut acts as an antiseptic.

Stings and bites Bee stings are acidic: apply a mixture of one half teaspoonful of baking soda to half a cup of water. Wasp stings are alkaline: apply cider vinegar or lemon juice. A raw onion and lavender oil will soothe both.

Burns Immerse in cold water for ten minutes. Break an aloe vera cacti leaf for a soothing gel. Dab on lavender oil (diluted with vegetable oil if necessary) or apply comfrey ointment.

Coughs Slice an onion in a deep bowl, cover with liquid honey, and leave overnight. The onion juice diffuses into the honey. Take a dessertspoonful of the mixture as needed.

Colds Ginger drink: slice 1 oz fresh ginger root and add 5 cloves, 2 broken cinnamon sticks, 1 teaspoon coriander seeds, and 1 pint water. Boil and simmer for 15 minutes, strain off herbs, add a squeeze of lemon juice and 1 teaspoon honey. Adults can add a tot of whisky or brandy.

Headaches Eat a piece of feverfew leaf between two slices of bread for migraine. Apply oil of rosemary to the head. Drink camomile tea for stress headaches.

NB *Always consult a doctor for severe symptoms or if the complaint does not improve within a few days.*

Doctors say

The medical profession is generally unacquainted with herbalism and, consequently, sceptical, although a number concede that many herbal remedies have fewer side effects than many conventional drugs.

Not all herbs are safe, however, and herbal medicine should not be taken without expert advice, especially if conventional medication is also being used.

Plants that should be avoided in pregnancy, as they may cause miscarriage, include motherwort or mugwort, golden seal, juniper, pennyroyal and pokeroot. Sage and marjoram are probably safe enough in cooking but not as herbal teas.

Rating

Popularity	Medical Credibility	Scientific Research	Availability
★★★★	★★★	★★★	★★★

HOMEOPATHY

In an old folk remedy, stinging nettles are used to treat painful joints swollen with rheumatism. This is the same 'like may be cured by like' principle on which homeopathy is based: a substance that causes certain symptoms in a healthy person can cure someone else who has developed similar symptoms as the result of disease. Arsenic, for example, much favoured by murder mystery writers for its promptness of despatch, is a common homeopathic remedy for diarrhoea and food poisoning.

Symptoms of disease – such as sore throat, fever, vomiting, inflammation – are signs that our body systems are fighting infection. Unlike orthodox medicine, in which you take a drug to reduce a fever, a homeopath will not try to suppress your symptoms, but will prescribe a remedy that, in normal doses, would produce similar effects – in fact, the closer the resemblance the better. This is to jolt our own self-healing powers, the so-called 'vital force', into action.

Despite using plant, mineral and animal substances such as arsenic and belladonna that in full-strength could kill you, homeopathic remedies are completely safe. This is because they are diluted thousands of times over until there are only a few molecules left, if any at all, of the original substance.

After each dilution, the mixture is shaken vigorously (known as *sucussion*) to transfer energy from the substance and *potentiate* its curative properties. The *weaker* the solution, therefore, the *more* effective homeopaths believe it to be. A decimal dilution of 6× equals one part in a million; roughly equivalent to a pinch of salt in a bath of water. On the centesimal scale, a 12c dilution is said to be comparable to a pinch of salt in the Atlantic Ocean.

How dilution works, nobody knows for sure. 'Does water have a memory?' science writers asked after a major research paper supporting homeopathy was published in 1988. The most popular theory is that the substance somehow leaves 'footprints' in the solution that the body recognises.

Because illness is considered to be the result of an inner imbalance, homeopaths take stock of the whole person: psychological, emotional and spiritual state of health as well as physical condition.

Every individual is unique, and the skill of the homeopathic practitioner lies in matching as many of your symptoms (*particulars*), habits (*generals*) and personality traits (*mentals*) to one of the two thousand or so remedies available. A cold, for instance, will be treated differently according to whether you are a jolly, overweight and outgoing person, or thin and neurotic.

Some remedies work well for everybody – arnica is universally used for shock and bruising – but certain types of people respond more strongly to particular substances. According to homeopath Dr Andrew Lockie, the people who react to, say, Natrum mur (derived from common salt) 'tend to be pear-shaped, have a dark complexion, be fastidious and rigid in personality, keep themselves to themselves, crave salt and suffer from constipation.'

The idea of 'similars' – treating like with like – had been around since the time of Hippocrates in the fourth century BC, but nobody paid much attention to it, until a German physician turned translator, Samuel Hahnemann, dosed himself with quinine and found that it produced the symptoms of malaria.

Intrigued, he persuaded healthy people to test – or 'prove' – other substances, such as arsenic, belladonna and mercury. The more he diluted the solution to make it safe, the stronger the response. In 1810 he published, *An Organon of Rational Healing*, explaining his theory of homeopathy from the Greek *omio*, meaning 'same', and *pathos*, 'suffering'.

Hahnemann's ideas spread from Germany throughout Europe to Asia and the Americas. In Britain, it became extremely fashionable; the first homeopathic hospital opened in London in 1850, and Queen Adelaide, consort to William IV, was the first of many members of the Royal Family to consult a homeopathic doctor.

The present Queen appoints a homeopathic physician to attend her, and apparently never travels far without what one Royal-watching journalist described as 'a battered black box full of medicines many chemists have never heard of'. This Royal backing goes a long way towards explaining why homeopathy, a system of medicine that defies current scientific explanation, can be prescribed on the NHS, and why there are five NHS homeopathic hospitals in the UK.

Best for

Homeopathy is not a suitable treatment in surgical emergencies or conditions such as cancer, although it has a supportive role. It is best for allergies, chronic conditions, digestive problems, some infections, some psychological disorders and women's health problems.

What happens

Because it is important for the homeopath to find out as much as possible about you and the type of person you are, the initial consultation can take up to an hour and a half. You will be asked detailed questions about your medical history, what you eat, your personal circumstances, your moods, any medication you are taking, and what your likes and dislikes are.

The homeopath will list your symptoms, compare them with those in the homeopath's prescribing handbook, and choose a remedy that fits your 'picture.' Remedies come as tablets, powders, granules, creams or drops. The homeopath may dispense the remedy, or you can buy it from a health shop or chemist. Less common remedies have to be purchased over the counter, or by mail order, from a homeopathic pharmacist.

You will also receive advice on your diet and lifestyle; cutting out coffee usually heads the list.

Olga remarks:

'Our son Buster, now four, was born prematurely with a lung infection. By the time he was 18 months old he had been quite ill, in and out of hospital several times, and he was always wheezy. Someone said "why not try homeopathy", so I did. I was very impressed by the questions the homeopath asked about Buster's background, his birth, his personality, his eating and sleeping habits. She gave me a remedy containing phosphorus, and later, when I read more about homeopathy,

I realised the personality described for it exactly fitted Buster's character.

'I first gave him the remedy the day we drove to the country for the weekend. By the time we arrived, he was very ill and wheezy with a temperature, and my husband was furious and accused me of practising witchcraft.

'I rang the homeopath when we got home, and she said "It sounds hard, but it's a good sign". After a week Buster was better – and for the first time in his life had stopped wheezing completely. My husband changed his mind about homeopathy!

'Since then he has had three or four attacks of asthma, with longer intervals between each. Of course we see the doctor, but I also go to the homeopath for a remedy. The rest of the time he is very healthy, eats well and doesn't have what they call an asthmatic chest.

'The homeopath treated our second son, Charlie, successfully when he suffered very badly from eczema as a baby. Occasionally it returns, very slightly, but clears up when he takes a remedy. I've been so convinced that I'm now studying to be homeopath myself.'

Self-help

Simple homeopathic remedies are available from health shops and chemists, such as Boots. Since a homeopath will prescribe a remedy tailor-made for you, over-the-counter remedies can be rather hit or miss. Manufacturers of hay fever remedies, for instance, will combine half a dozen substances in the hope there will be something to suit everyone. If you buy them, follow the instructions for dosage on the label carefully, and consult a good reference book.

A good standby in the medicine cabinet, because it works for everyone, is *arnica*, the universal remedy for shock, falls, bruising, bleeding, exhaustion and jet lag.

Doctors say

Although this is the most mainstream of complementary therapies and available on the NHS, homeopathy is not yet taught in medical schools, and many doctors have problems with the idea that the more a remedy is diluted, the more effective it is.

None the less the number of GPs interested in homeopathy is growing, especially if they are young and/or female. According to a survey by *Doctor* in 1992, 80 per cent of GPs who responded believed homeopathy was effective.

Among sceptics, relief from symptoms is often attributed to the placebo effect (the idea that a treatment works because the patient believes it will), but several clinical trials at the NHS Glasgow Homeopathic Hospital in the 1980s showed that, even allowing for this effect, homeopathic remedies successfully alleviated rheumatoid arthritis and hay fever.

There was great excitement in 1988 when a series of experiments by Jacques Benveniste seemed to show some kind of change in water in which a substance had been diluted to the point of disappearance. This controversy is still unresolved.

Rating

Popularity	Medical Credibility	Scientific Research	Availability
✯✯✯✯	✯✯✯	✯✯✯✯	✯✯✯✯

HYDROTHERAPY

Most people's idea of water therapy is a relaxing soak in a fragrant bath or a shower to freshen up. The gentle pummelling of water jets in a jacuzzi is lovely, and it is hard to beat a splash in the sea for invigoration.

The healing and cleansing properties of water have been acknowledged for many centuries. The Greeks believed it contained the essence of life and the secret of health, and no Roman town was complete without its baths, where citizens could pass the time of day while moving between hot bath, cold bath and tepid bath.

It grew very fashionable to 'take the waters' at natural hot mineral springs, such as Bath in Britain, Baden-Baden in Germany and Spa in Belgium. But serious hydrotherapy had to wait until Vincent

Priessnitz, an Austrian, opened a spa at Grafenberg, in the early nineteenth century. As part of his rigorous regime, buckets of icy cold water were emptied on patients from such a height they had to clutch a supporting bar.

A Bavarian monk, Father Sebastian Kneipp (1821–1897), refined this process. He claimed water could cure every disease by dissolving the toxins and expelling them from the body. He put patients through a programme of hot and cold baths, vapour baths, showers, foot baths, hot and cold compresses, sitz baths (in which you sit in a hot bath with your feet in a cold one, and then reverse the procedure) and wrapping. In the latter, still offered by some naturopathic spas for skin disorders, colds, bronchitis and back pain, patients are wrapped in a cold wet sheet, then a dry sheet and a warm blanket, left until the wet sheet has dried out, then sponged with tepid water and dried.

Turkish baths, steam baths and saunas, popular in health farms and clubs, gently cook you until you perspire and impurities are flushed out through the open pores of the skin. The latest vogue in health farms is *thalassatherapy*, or sea-water treatment, following the discovery of a link between the mineral salts in our blood and those in the sea.

Alexandra, a health and beauty writer who visited a French thalassatherapy spa in the line of duty, related:

'I never realised there are a hundred different ways of bathing in sea water. In one treatment, we took off our clothes and stood in a tiled room, while a woman stood four feet away and turned what seemed to be a fireman's hose on us. Then I was wrapped in seaweed, went to sleep, woke up to have a bubbling sea-water bath, a massage with seaweed cream, and made to do exercises in a pool against underwater jets. I have to say that it was unbelievably relaxing, like a week at the seaside compressed into one day, and I felt wonderful.'

Best for

A host of complaints respond to this therapy, including back pain, joint problems, rheumatism, muscular strains, arthritis, asthma, menstrual problems, anxiety and fatigue. Physiotherapists take patients suffering disability, or recovering from stroke or injury, into a warm pool for exercise, relaxation and massage.

Doctors say

Apart from physiotherapy, most doctors are unlikely to recommend anything more than a weekend in a health farm, a holiday by the sea or regular swimming. Those allergic to iodine should avoid seaweed treatments, and anyone suffering from heart disease or high blood pressure should consult a doctor before any treatment involving hot and/or cold water temperatures.

Rating

Popularity	Medical Credibility	Scientific Research	Availability
☆☆	☆☆☆	☆☆	☆☆☆

HYPNOTHERAPY

Hypnotherapy has suffered from a bad press – too many showmen swinging fobwatches, too many stagey hypnotists, too many stories of Svengalis taking advantage of defenceless young women. Too much quackery, too many charlatans.

The irony is that more scientific evidence exists to back hypnotherapy than almost any other complementary therapy. It is a convincing demonstration of the power of the mind over the body.

You really *can* put somebody into a trance and make suggestions to them that they will later carry out. In this peculiar 'hypnogogic' state, somewhere between waking and sleeping, when utterly relaxed, focused and extraordinarily receptive, people can perform prodigious feats of strength and memory, of will power and self-healing.

Nobody yet understands how this is achieved, although some believe the hypnotherapist is bypassing the patient's conscious left brain hemisphere, the seat of reasoning and critical judgement, and tapping the right brain's intuitive and creative powers.

It is claimed that nine out of ten people can be hypnotised by a skilled hypnotist, as can the remaining tenth, if an appropriate method is used. A sleep-inducing environment may do the trick: motorway drivers have reported a trance-like blanking out.

Much also depends on the co-operation and willingness (conscious or unconscious) of the subject and the personal rapport with the hypnotist. The best hypnotic subjects are those who are easily absorbed in what they are doing; the most difficult are those who are readily distracted, active and analytical. Women often make better subjects than men.

In a *light* trance, the eyes are closed, you feel deeply relaxed and prepared to accept ego-boosting suggestions, such as 'I am confident and easy in new situations.'

Most therapy takes place in a *medium* trance, when heartbeat, respiration and metabolism are slowed, and brainwave frequencies are similar to those in meditation. You feel less pain (dentists practising hypnotherapy work at this level), and allergic reactions stop.

Only ten per cent of the population can readily be taken into a *deep* trance. This is the real sleepwalking state; the eyes are open and yet minor operations can be performed without anaesthesia, and people regress into infancy.

The ancient Egyptians and Greeks, and tribal cultures in Africa and North America, obviously had some knowledge of hypnotic techniques in inducing altered states of consciousness, but the generally accepted founder of modern hypnotism is a German physician, Franz Mesmer. Through a process he called 'animal magnetism', he could induce a loss of mental and physical control in his patients.

'Animal magnetism' was ultimately rejected as worthless, but his followers discovered that if those in a trance were told they could feel no pain, then no pain was felt. Research into what was now called 'hypnosis' was going well, led by a Scot, surgeon James Braid, when the anaesthetic properties of ether were discovered and medical science took a different course. Hypnosis was pushed to the sideline, where it languished until American psychologists in the

1930s put the research spotlight on it again, this time as a drug-free relaxant that was useful in treating stress-related disorders.

Best for

Stress-related conditions such as anxiety, asthma, insomnia, migraine, irritable bowel syndrome, gastric ulcer, colitis, constipation, allergies; eczema, warts, psoriasis and other skin complaints; pain relief, especially during labour and dental treatment; menstrual disorders; addictions and habits such as eating disorders, smoking and alcohol dependency; fears, phobias, lack of confidence, inhibitions, and sexual problems. More recently, it has been used for the relief of suffering and depression in those undergoing acute medical treatment and those who are terminally ill.

What happens

It is important to have trust in your hypnotherapist, and some people might feel more comfortable with a practitioner of the same sex. The hypnotherapist should ask about your physical and mental health, and your particular problem – whether there are any deeper causes, and how motivated you are about resolving it.

Practitioners use different methods to induce a trance. You will be encouraged to lie back on a reclining chair or couch, while the practitioner talks slowly and soothingly, guiding your mind into a concentrated and detached state. You may be asked to visualise a walk in the country, or to look at lights or a pencil held at the limits of vision, or the practitioner may repeat a monotonous series of statements.

It will be suggested to you that you feel heavy and your eyes are closing, and your hand is growing lighter and rising. If it does, you are already in a light trance. For a deeper trace, the practitioner might count you down to ten, or ask you to imagine yourself descending in a lift.

Some hypnotists then plant the suggestion that the symptom is going ('You never want to smoke again.') and make encouraging statements about feeling positive and self-confident. A hypnotist trained in medicine or psychotherapy however, will want to go further and deal with the root of the problem, helping you to change your attitude or examine underlying feelings of guilt, anger or fear. In trained hands, hypnotherapy is a wonderful tool for pinpointing the long-buried childhood traumas that are the source of present pain.

Lucy, a public relations consultant with a five-year-old son, said:

'Recurring nightmares took me to a hypnotherapist about three years ago. I felt slightly apprehensive – I don't want people messing with my mind unless I trust them – but it all seemed quite straightforward; I sat down, she asked me some questions, not too self-revealing, and then I lay down on the sofa and closed my eyes. She spoke very gently and I felt myself drifting away. I can't remember the core details now, but I know she talked about safety and confidence. It was very soothing, and it has been a bit of a help. I've had fewer nightmares since, although I think it might be even more effective if used with other therapies.'

You may be taught techniques of self-hypnosis to manage your condition in daily living. Phobics and asthmatics, for example, can learn to relax and control an attack before it has time to take hold.

Are there risks in hypnotherapy? Generally not. Hypnotherapists say you cannot be hypnotised against your will, nor made to do anything that you do not wish to do. Most practitioners are sensible about post-hypnotic suggestions, but a strong argument for choosing a practitioner with a training in psychotherapy is the possibility that a more serious physical or psychological condition might be uncovered.

Neither can one entirely rule out the risk of manipulation or sexual, emotional or financial abuse; another reason to make sure you trust your practitioner. There has been considerable controversy in the UK and US recently over 'false memory', where people claim to recall incidents of childhood sexual abuse. Sceptics believe that these could be 'planted', perhaps unwittingly, in suggestible subjects.

Doctors say

Poorly trained and manipulative hypnotherapists give cause for concern, and the profession needs to organise training standards, registration, and a code of ethics as soon as possible. Used responsibly, hypnotherapy is an asset. Much research has shown that, at the very least, it can induce relaxation, relieve anxiety and alter mood. Studies have demonstrated numerous other effects: in one trial hypnotherapy eased irritable bowel syndrome, and, in another, children using chemotherapy vomited less and maintained a higher fluid intake when taught self-hypnosis.

Rating

Popularity	Medical Credibility	Scientific Research	Availability
✮✮✮✮	✮✮✮✮	✮✮✮✮	✮✮✮✮

IRIDOLOGY

The iris of the eye, according to iridologists, reflects the state of your physical and mental health. From its colouring, condition and markings, they claim to diagnose not only current and past disorders but give advance warning of what may come; an attractive proposition for anyone wary of conventional medical tests – blood samples, X-rays and barium meals.

The iris is said to represent a body map, divided into sections representing different parts and systems – the kidney, for example is a segment at the bottom, the lymphatic and circulatory systems lie in an outer ring. The left eye, say iridologists, corresponds to the left hand side of the body, the right to the right-hand side. White marks on the iris are said to show signs of stress and inflammation in the relevant organ; black marks indicate a malfunction. The dark rim around the iris of many smokers, according to practitioners, reveals the accumulation of toxins in the body.

Modern iridology, also called ophthalmic somatology, began in the mid-nineteenth century with a Hungarian doctor, Ignatz von Peczely, who, as a boy, tended an owl with a broken leg, and noticed a black mark in the bird's eye that changed as its leg healed. In 1950, an American physician, Dr Bernard Jensen, constructed the map of the iris which is now the basis of diagnosis.

What happens

Initial consultations usually last about an hour, and fees range from £40. Practioners of another therapy, such as naturopathy or herbalism, who use iridology as an extra diagnostic tool, examine the iris with a torch and magnifying glass, and make a drawing. A specialist iridologist will use a camera with close-up lens and side-lighting to make a photographic slide of the eye, which is then projected on to a screen for detailed examination. According to the conditions identified, you will be referred to an appropriate practitioner or to your GP.

Doctors say

The general appearance of the eye, its brightness or the colour of the white, *can* be a rough guide to health, but most orthodox doctors would regard the idea that the iris is a detailed map of the body with scepticism.

Rating

Popularity	Medical Credibility	Scientific Research	Availability
☆☆☆	☆☆	☆☆☆	☆☆

KINESIOLOGY

Whether your limb holds firm or sags when pressure is applied to muscles in your arm or leg can tell a kinesiologist your state of health. From this response, practitioners claim to diagnose blockages and imbalances in the functioning of the body systems, your emotional condition, or whether you are allergic to certain foods.

While working on a patient with severe leg pains in 1964, George Goodheart, an American chiropractor, discovered that massaging a certain muscle alleviated the pain. As a result, he developed a system known as Applied Kinesiology, based on the idea that each group of muscles is related to other, often distant, parts of the body.

Kinesiologists refer to an invisible energy, comparable to an electric current, that runs in circuits through the body – so we have the 'kidney circuit' or the 'pancreas circuit'. These correspond exactly to the twelve classical *meridians* of Chinese medicine, and the energy to Qi, the life force (see *Acupuncture, Traditional Chinese Medicine*).

Practitioners unblock and rebalance the circuits by applying finger tip massage to 'pressure points', that happen to be in the same position as acupressure points. This is said to restore blood circulation and the flow of lymph, a body fluid that drains toxins from the tissues.

Many chiropractors and osteopaths now use kinesiology, especially in the US and Australia, and it is increasingly popular in international sports medicine.

More controversial, however, is its use in allergy testing. Foods and substances suspected of interfering with the body's electrical field are placed in the hand, on the body (i.e. stomach) or under the tongue, and the muscles tested for response.

Abi, a young woman with an allergy to dairy products, said:

> *'The kinesiologist put a tiny crumb of cheese under my tongue and immediately my arm gave way when he put gentle pressure on it. Only seconds before I'd been able to resist him.'*

Best for

Allergies and food sensitivities, leading to colds, depression, headaches, fatigue and weaknesses in the immune system; the identification of vitamin and mineral deficiencies; back pain and neck pain. Many practitioners diagnose and treat weaknesses in the body systems, without paying too much attention to specific symptoms.

What happens

You will be asked about your medical history and general health, before sitting or lying on a treatment couch. The practitioner may want your legs and arms bare for testing, so be prepared to take some garments off unless wearing light summer clothes.

Major muscle groups will be tested first. You will be asked to hold your arm or leg in a certain position, while the practitioner presses gently for a few seconds to test your ability to exert an opposite pressure. If your limb feels 'spongy', further touch tests will be done to find out why, then the practitioner will gently brush along the meridians to unblock the energy flow.

If you are being tested for allergies, you will be given a series of substances either to hold in your hand or put under your tongue while muscle response is tested.

Initial consultations last about an hour, and you should feel an immediate sense of well-being, although further visits may be necessary. Fees range from £15 to £30 per session.

Doctors say

There is a lack of scientific research, although a number of doctors are beginning to use kinesiology to help diagnosis. Many are open-minded, but some conventional practitioners regard it as dressing up traditional Chinese medicine concepts of Qi in Westernised terms of electrical currents.

Rating

Popularity	Medical Credibility	Scientific Research	Availability
✲✲✲	✲✲	✲✲	✲✲✲

LIGHT THERAPY (PHOTOTHERAPY)

Seasonal Affective Disorder (SAD) is the name given to severe winter blues. Linked to sun and daylight starvation, sufferers' mood droops as days shorten in autumn, and remains depressed until the longer days of spring. Many complain of persistent tiredness, lethargy and food bingeing.

Increased levels of the hormone melatonin in the bloodstream have been found responsible for this depression. Melatonin induces drowsiness, affecting our daily rhythms of sleep and mood. It is secreted by the pineal gland at the base of the brain, which is stimulated by light entering through the eyes. At night when it is time to sleep, melatonin levels rise, and, at dawn, daylight prompts the gland to stop production so that we become active.

People suffering from SAD (an estimated one per cent of the population, and four times as many women as men), have difficulty training their pineal glands to adapt to the lack of morning light in winter.

The average intensity of daylight is 5000 lux (the unit of illuminance), and indoor light is only 500 lux. Light therapy, in which sufferers sit beside a light box emitting 2500 lux for a couple of hours a day, seems sufficient to influence hormone production, and is successful for about 80 per cent of sufferers.

Best for
Those suffering from SAD, premenstrual tension and sleeping difficulty; also nightshift workers.

Doctors say
There is now a body of research, mainly from North America, which has studied the influence of light on hormone production. Many of those using light therapy say that it alleviates their seasonal depression. In short, it can do no harm, and it may do some good.

Rating

Popularity	Medical Credibility	Scientific Research	Availability
☆	☆☆	☆☆	☆

MASSAGE

'Let me rub it better,' mothers instinctively say to children when they fall over and graze their knees. To stroke someone in anguish, rub a part of the body that hurts, or clutch oneself in despair, is the most natural thing in the world. This intuitive response is the earliest and simplest form of massage, an ancient therapy – if not the most ancient – that Western medicine is now rediscovering.

Massage is the kneading and stroking with the hands of the body's soft tissues – the skin and muscles – with varying degrees of pressure. Done gently, it affects the nervous system, and brings a therapeutic feeling of relaxation and comfort. Nerve endings that respond to pain as well as touch are in the skin, and it is thought that stimulating the latter can somehow release endorphins and reduce sensations of pain.

Stronger massage stimulates the blood circulation and lymphatic (or waste drainage) systems of the body, easing knotted tissues, relaxing muscles and clearing away toxins that can crystallise in the tissues and cause pain and stiffness. This in turn improves breathing and digestion. Massage is not a cure for any specific complaint, but the sense of invigoration and well-being that results can help prevent disease by dispelling the stress hormones that weaken the immune system.

Egyptian tomb paintings show people having their feet massaged, and the ancient Greek and Roman physicians regarded massage as one of the principle methods of healing and relieving pain. Hippocrates, the father of medicine, wrote in the fifth century BC: 'The physician must be experienced in many things, but assuredly in rubbing… For rubbing can bind a joint that is too loose, and loosen a joint that is too rigid.' The way to health, he added, was a scented bath and an oiled massage every day.

In the West, massage has fallen in and out of favour over the centuries, largely due to the Christian Church's ambivalent attitude towards anything that seemed to indulge the body. (Many people today still regard massage as a luxury.) Ambroise Paré, physician to the sixteenth century French court, sang the praises of massage in treating various ailments, but it was Per Henrik Ling, a Swedish gymnast in the early part of the nineteenth century, who put therapeutic massage on the medical map again.

His 'Swedish movement treatment', grounded in anatomy, is the basis for the techniques used in modern Western massage. The most common movements you will encounter include *effleurage*, a light, firm and gentle stroking; *petrissage*, a firm kneading and rolling of the tissues; and *tapotement,* hacking, tapping and clapping over the muscles and fleshy parts of the body.

St Thomas's Hospital in London had a department of massage until 1934, and physiotherapy is based on Ling's massage methods, but, as a therapy, massage was forgotten in the excitement of new health care technology after the war. At the same time, the term acquired undesirable associations with seedy massage parlours and prostitution. The words 'masseur' and 'masseuse' have such a derogatory connotation that practitioners prefer to call themselves massage practitioners or even bodywork practitioners.

However, serious massage is now making a comeback, largely through the nursing profession which has always acknowledged the healing qualities of touch. Clare Maxwell-Hudson, the pioneering massage practitioner who runs one of Britain's top schools of massage training, has led teams of practitioners into NHS hospitals for more than twelve years, and now teaches massage to degree students at the Royal College of Nursing. Advanced massage is a module in the new Masters degree in Therapeutic Bodywork at the University of Westminster.

Clare Maxwell-Hudson said recently:

> *'Many nurses tell me that massage enables them to feel they are offering proper nursing again, rather than giving pills. In order for people to become well, it's essential for them to be able to relax. Anxiety and tension can prolong illness.'*

In NHS hospitals, massage is used in intensive care units, for children and elderly people, for babies in incubators, and cancer, AIDS, heart attack and stroke patients. Some GP surgeries, drug dependency clinics, pain clinics and hospices also offer massage.

Ordinary people can learn simple massage to comfort relatives who are sick or dying. At one London hospital, patients suffering from severe constipation and irritable bowel syndrome are taught self-massage techniques, a more effective treatment than laxatives or enemas.

Massage techniques are also used in a number of complementary therapies, notably *aromatherapy, reflexology, polarity therapy, kinesiology* and *shiatsu.* There are several styles of massage available, and practitioners frequently use a combination. *Swedish massage* is found in health spas and sports clubs and among aromatherapists and massage practitioners. *Eastern massage*, as in shiatsu, works on balancing the energy forces in the body. *Holistic massage* takes into account the emotional needs of the receiver as well as the physical, and has a strong intuitive element. *Remedial massage* concentrates on specific conditions, such as muscle strains.

Best for

Relaxation and stress-related conditions, such as insomnia and headaches, especially when part of a total stress-management programme. It is also used to treat asthma, rheumatism, constipation, irritable bowel syndrome, depression, and high blood pressure, and to relieve arthritis, backache, joint sprains, muscular strain and sciatica. In sports medicine, massage is used to help athletes prepare for competition and ease muscle tensions.

What happens

Therapeutic massage is available at some GP surgeries, drug dependency clinics, pain clinics and hospices. Health farms and clubs, sports centres and beauty clinics routinely offer massage, and private practitioners will come to your home or even workplace, for an on-site neck and shoulder massage at your desk.

At the first visit, you will be asked briefly about your medical history, lifestyle and general state of health. Mention any medication you are taking, and try not to eat or drink too heavily beforehand. Massage is not recommended if you suffer from phlebitis (vein inflammation), thrombosis, varicose veins, tumours, acute back pain or fever of any kind, or if you are in the first three months of pregnancy. In later pregnancy, only gentle massage is advised. Any swellings, skin infections or bruises will be avoided. If you have any doubts, check beforehand with your GP.

For a whole body massage, it is usual to undress, although some people prefer to keep on their underpants. During the massage (which is generally on a massage table, but can be given on a futon mattress or thick blanket on the floor) towels are folded over you, to keep you warm as much as to preserve your dignity.

The back is usually treated first, followed by the neck and legs. Then you turn over and the front of the legs, shoulders, arms and hands, neck and face are massaged. Individual practitioners have slightly different ways of working, but a professional practitioner's manner should relieve any embarrassment. You do not have to converse; apart from comments about possible areas of discomfort, many practitioners prefer to work in silence so they can attune themselves to your body.

When the massage is finished, you will be left alone for a few moments to savour the after-glow. You should feel warm and relaxed. Some people may find massage arouses feelings of sadness or lightheadedness, and others may ache a little the next day.

A whole body massage lasts about an hour and a half, and expect to pay from £20 to £40, depending on where you live.

Doctors say
The benefits of massage are becoming so obvious that few would argue with them. In some recent research studies, premature babies massaged over ten days gained weight faster and were sent home earlier than those not massaged, and elderly people given massage in addition normal conversation reported lower anxiety scores than those having conversation only sessions.

Rating

Popularity	Medical Credibility	Scientific Research	Availability
★★★★	★★★★	★★★	★★★★

MEDITATION

Meditation has suffered a rather cranky image in the Western press, ever since the Beatles took off to India in pursuit of the Maharishi Mahesh Yogi. But the practice is not confined to orange-garbed followers of Eastern gurus, cross-legged in the lotus position, silently intoning 'Om'.

Long before the Maharishi's Transcendental Meditation (TM), hit the West, people in the Christian and Jewish mystic traditions practised meditation. Fourteenth-century Christian writers refer to withdrawing from ordinary consciousness to contact God, and the Byzantine Church used the repetitive Jesus Prayer, or Prayer of the Heart, 'Lord Jesus Christ, have mercy on me'.

You do not have to be religious to meditate – although when it becomes a regular habit it can lead to spiritual development. Those who have meditated for years speak of attaining moments of profound bliss and fulfilment.

Physiologically and psychologically, it is good for your health. American researchers, particularly Dr Herbert Benson of the Harvard Medical School, showed that meditation decreases the blood pressure and breathing rate, slows the heartbeat and lowers the metabolic rate to levels not found outside very deep sleep or hibernation. The brainwave frequency changes to the long alpha waves that are a sign of deep relaxation coupled with a state of mental alertness.

Far from being woolly and otherworldly, regular meditators seem to have greater powers of concentration and a sense of control over their lives that enables them to be extraordinarily efficient. Dr Benson speaks of a mental plasticity that he called 'the Principle of Maximum Mind', or being receptive to new ways of seeing the world and ourselves.

Schools of meditation lay down rules about how you should sit, or what mental exercises to perform, but Dr Benson found that anybody could achieve this state of relaxed awareness provided they followed four basic rules:

- a quiet environment;

- a comfortable position, usually sitting so as to prevent sleep or drowsiness;

- an object for the attention to dwell on (such as the breath or a mantra, the repetition of a particular word or phrase) so that the flood of information and sensations rushing around our heads can be ignored;

- passive awareness. This is the most difficult concept to get across to Western minds accustomed to constant busyness, but it is a kind of mindfulness, noting what passes through your attention but letting things be.

Best for

Anybody interested in personal development. Healthwise, it benefits those suffering from high blood pressure, chronic pain, tension headaches, chilblains and Raynaud's disease (because it improves circulation), asthma, insomnia and other stress-related problems.

How to meditate

- Find a place where you will not be disturbed.

- Make sure the room is warm and your clothes comfortable.

- If you can, practise for fifteen or twenty minutes twice a day, before a meal. Set a clock or kitchen timer so you need not worry about the time.

- A cross-legged lotus pose is not necessary. Sit on an upright chair, back comfortably straight, feet firmly on the ground, hands in your lap or on your knees, palms either up or down. Imagine a straight line aligning your navel with the tip of your nose, or a string pulling you up from the crown of your head. Close your eyes and relax.

- Breathe rhymthmically and slowly through your nose and down into your abdomen.

- Focus on the object of your meditation. It could be your breath, watching it go in and out as you count to four; or an image, real or imaginary, to hold in your mind – a candleflame or a flower; or a word or phrase to repeat. Many people use 'peace' or 'one'.

- When your mind wanders, bring it gently back to the object of meditation; there is no need to be anxious.

- At the end, take a full minute to come back slowly to everyday life. Open your eyes and become fully aware of your surroundings. Stretch, and move your arms and legs about before getting up. Your blood pressure will have dropped, so do not stand up quickly.

Doctors say

The benefits of meditation, both physically and emotionally, are well documented, although there is now some evidence that it is possible for some people to meditate to excess, so that they become too relaxed and too plastic, and they either withdraw from real life or become emotionally raw.

Rating

Popularity	Medical Credibility	Scientific Research	Availability
✮✮✮✮	✮✮✮	✮✮✮✮	✮✮✮✮

METAMORPHIC TECHNIQUE

According to practitioners, the foot reflects the body's development in the womb, when the physical, mental and emotional patterns of our lives are established, and future responses to disease indicated.

By gently stroking and massaging the feet, hands and head, they claim people can come to terms with tensions in the body and mind, especially those determined before birth.

Developed in the 1960s by a British naturopath, Robert St John, from his work with reflexology, the technique makes no claims to cure, but tries to help people develop a more positive approach that will encourage them to take creative steps to change their life.

Best for

Those with long-standing health problems, including physically and mentally handicapped people.

What happens

Practitioners describe themselves not as practitioners, but catalysts (agents of change), and therefore remain detached throughout the treatment, offering no response or counselling. You sit comfortably while each foot is manipulated in turn with light circular strokes, followed by the hands and head. The feet are said to represent movement and energy, the hands action, the head thought. As each is touched, old ways of behaving and thinking are loosened and new ones allowed to surface.

Expect to pay at least £20 for a session, which usually lasts about an hour. These take place weekly until you feel ready to cope on your own. The practitioner will offer to teach the basic technique to a member of your family, so that you can continue the process at home.

Doctors say
This is a non-invasive treatment that people may well find helpful. As usual, any symptoms of ill health should be referred to your GP.

Rating

Popularity	Medical Credibility	Scientific Research	Availability
☆	☆☆	☆	☆

MUSIC THERAPY

'Everyone who plays an instrument or listens to music for pleasure knows that music has potent effects upon mind and body,' wrote psychiatrist Anthony Storr. 'Music can alter our moods, reduce fatigue, facilitate muscular movement, stir our memories.'

The link between music and healing has been acknowledged for thousands of years. In the Old Testament, David played the harp to King Saul when he was possessed of an evil spirit, and 'the spirit departed from him'. Making music, too, allows us to express emotions – anger, sorrow, longing, joy – that may be too profound and too primitive for mere words.

As a creative expression, music therapy is opening doors for those who are mentally and emotionally disabled. The therapist will start by playing a tune or song, and gradually, as the patient responds, they communicate and make music together, often improvising with drums and percussion instruments.

Best for
Music therapy has benefited autistic children and others with mental handicap, physical disabilities and emotional disturbances; those with eating disorders and the elderly. It can also relieve stress and anxiety, pain, depression and helplessness.

Doctors say
The benefits of music therapy are now widely recognised, and it is used with growing frequency in the NHS. Current research is investigating the effects of music on the brain; one recent study showed that listening to music increased a factor of the immune system which can be detected in saliva.

Rating

Popularity	Medical Credibility	Scientific Research	Availability
☆☆☆	☆☆☆	☆☆☆	☆☆☆

NATUROPATHY

If you have a fever, a naturopath would advise you not to take a temperature-reducing drug, such as aspirin or paracetamol, but to sweat it out. As one practitioner put it: 'The body lights a fire inside that burns out the toxins, and it shouldn't be suppressed.'

Naturopathy – also known as natural medicine, nature cure and natural therapeutics – is based on a belief that the body has the ability to heal itself: *vis medicatrix naturae* – the healing power of nature.

Illness is said to result from a weakening of the individual's 'vital force', when viruses, bacteria and allergens may take hold. This weakness is blamed on an accumulation of waste products, toxins and other rubbish caused by a deficient lifestyle: too much stress, food loaded with chemicals, environmental pollution and not enough fresh air and exercise.

Rather than knock out the disease with drugs, a naturopath will work towards identifying the underlying cause of the symptoms, and then set about finding ways of restoring your inner self-regulating harmony, known as 'homeostasis'.

If the body can heal cuts or mend broken bones, naturopaths point out, then it can probably deal with other disorders. This natural healing process is begun by ridding the body of toxins and bolstering its defences.

Symptoms such as fever are signs that the body is calling on its self-healing powers, and – so long as the situation is not life-threatening – should be left to get on with the job. When symptoms are suppressed, it is argued, disorders 'go underground,' becoming chronic and leading to further degeneration. The glue ear that plagues modern children might be an example: dosed with antibiotics as soon as they develop an ear infection, the mucus that blocks the tubes of the ear is never totally cleared, more infections follow, and finally the ear is so full of muck that hearing is affected and an operation is needed to drain it. A naturopath, on the other hand, would try to rectify the underlying catarrhal disorder.

Naturopathy is the Western version of other holistic nature-based medical systems that rely on herbal remedies and diet management, such as *Traditional Chinese Medicine* and *Ayurvedic Medicine* (see separate entries for these); the 'vital force' being comparable to the Chinese *Qi*.

Hippocrates, the father of medicine, laid the guidelines for naturopathy 2500 years ago. Health, he said, can be maintained by the correct balance of rest and exercise and plain food in moderation, and cures should be as natural as possible.

But the therapy really came into its own last century with the popularity of water cures and spa towns in Germany, where the nature-cure movement is still very much alive. Benedict Lust, one of the followers of Father Sebastian Kneipp, a Bavarian monk who launched health farms as we know them, took naturopathy to the

United States, where it blossomed and now includes nutritional therapies of every kind.

Best for

Naturopaths believe they can help a wide range of disorders, but naturopathy is said to be particularly effective with skin problems, asthma, allergies, premenstrual syndrome, rheumatoid arthritis, emphysema, ulcers and other gastrointestinal disorders.

What happens

Because the naturopath takes a holistic approach and wants to build a complete picture of each individual's life, the first consultation will last 45 to 60 minutes (expect to pay £30 to £50, depending on where you live, and less thereafter). You will be asked detailed questions, not only about your medical history, but your eating and sleeping patterns, bowel movements, menstrual cycle, work, relationships, likes and dislikes.

The practitioner will probably give you a routine medical examination, including blood pressure, lungs and heart, spinal joints and body reflexes, and may also arrange X-rays, blood and urine tests, and specialised scans such as ultrasound. Your irises may be examined (*iridology*) and blood, sweat or hair analysed for any mineral imbalances or toxic metal accumulations. If any condition requiring surgery or other treatments beyond the naturopath's expertise is uncovered, you would be referred to your GP.

When the underlying problem causing your symptoms has been diagnosed, the naturopath will make various suggestions about changing your lifestyle. The most common is to change your diet. You could be told to avoid dairy and wheat products if a food intolerance is suspected; or to eat more salads and cut out caffeine.

Sometimes fasting is recommended to detoxify the system. This could be three to five days on nothing but water, or (if you are lucky) fruit or vegetable juices.

Naturopaths are also trained in *hydrotherapy* and often in other disciplines, such as *osteopathy*, *acupuncture*, *herbalism*, and *homeopathy*, and may call on some of these treatments.

The length of treatment depends on your progress, and the naturopath will watch for various signs. Your health should steadily improve, punctuated by relapses known as 'healing crises.' When symptoms reappear, it will be in the reverse order of their appearance, like a tape unwinding, and the disease will move from the inside, from deep tissues and vital organs, to external ones like the skin. The last step on the road to good health could be a rash.

Doctors say

The principles of naturopathy are those of good health care, both as prevention and cure. All symptoms should be checked with your GP, however, to rule out any condition requiring surgery or other emergency measures, before embarking on a naturopathic regime.

Rating

Popularity	Medical Credibility	Scientific Research	Availability
✶✶✶✶	✶✶✶	✶✶✶	✶✶✶✶

NUTRITIONAL THERAPY

We are what we eat, or, in some cases, don't eat. Although the importance of nourishment in maintaining health has always been acknowledged, the link between what we swallow and its effects on our body is now of fast-expanding and (literally) consuming interest. 'Healthy eating' features in headlines everywhere.

More and more research studies highlight the role of, say, vitamin E in preventing heart disease, or that of antioxidant vitamins and minerals in combating cancer. Experts debate the influence of food additives on children's behaviour, and people discover that sometimes their fatigue, headaches and skin problems can be traced to certain foods.

Almost daily there is a story about nutrition in the press to add to the confusion. Fats are bad for you. Some fats are good for you. Eat more fibre to prevent colon cancer. Too much fibre can interfere with the body's absorption of iron. Alcohol causes cancer. A glass of wine prevents heart disease.

Theories and diets of every sort abound, from food combining to megavitamin doses and detoxifying coffee enemas. The shelves of health stores teem with bottles and packets of food supplements – vitamins, minerals, micronutrients, enzymes, herbs. Who can tell what is for the best?

Naturopathy has always emphasised the importance of plain food, unadorned with additives, preservatives and pesticides, and *clinical ecology* studies the ways that environmental factors can affect our diet and health. Nutritional therapy (or complementary nutritional therapy as it is sometimes known) tries to explore all possible avenues whereby the individual's self-healing process can be restored by adjusting their food and supplement intake.

Nutritional therapist Linda Lazarides, who is also secretary of the Society for the Promotion of Nutritional Therapy:

> *'People can have nutritional deficiencies even on a good diet. They might have food allergies that cause inflammation and malabsorption in the stomach, preventing nutrients getting into the bloodstream. Or even when the blood is full of nutrients, toxic overload, due to heavy metals or chemicals in the environment, can block absorption at a cellular level.'*

Best for
Nutritional therapists claim that few people with health problems would not benefit from the therapy, particularly those suffering from migraine, irritable bowel syndrome, chronic fatigue and skin or joint problems.

What happens
At the first consultation, the therapist will want to know about your health problem, and usually asks you to complete an exhaustive questionnaire about your medical history, symptoms, early life, lifestyle and typical food intake over three days. You should be advised to consult your GP as well, since nutritional therapists are not qualified in medical diagnosis, and would only claim to give 'health promotion advice'.

Expect to have explained how long and how expensive the therapy will be. Average fees are £20 to £40 an hour, and the therapist will probably want to see you every fortnight for about ten weeks, while 'therapeutic trials' are conducted. According to your complaint, various diets will be tried out and adjusted.

At the beginning some will seem rather radical, particularly detoxifying and semi-macrobiotic regimes, and Linda Lazarides admits that a lot of counselling and motivating may be needed to encourage people to continue. 'I say "It's not for a lifetime, try it for two weeks and see what happens" and they usually feel better, so they come back.'

As well as enzyme and herb remedies, high levels of vitamin and mineral supplements are sometimes recommended, but not in the megadoses popular in the US. At the end of the course, a less extreme maintenance diet will be established.

Doctors say

No one with a health problem should embark on a diet or course of supplements without consulting their doctor. Some nutritional supplements can interact with prescribed medication. High doses of vitamin C, for example, can reduce the effects of some anti-coagulants, and exacerbate the side effects of some antibiotics, and may contribute to the formation of kidney stones in susceptible people. In a 1990 Swedish study into deaths and complications from 'alternative' therapies, it was found that the majority of deaths occurred when patients whose diseases drew on their body's reserves were put on vegetarian diets or fasted.

Rating

Popularity	Medical Credibility	Scientific Research	Availability
✫✫✫	✫✫✫	✫✫✫	✫✫

OSTEOPATHY

Our bones and muscles are not merely some kind of coathanger for our heart and intestines. We have a 'moving' body, and life is what we do with it: walking, talking, running, climbing, building, loving – as well as breathing, digesting and eliminating.

Osteopathy has been called the science of human mechanics. Our musculo-skeletal system – bones, joints, muscles, ligaments and connective tissue – consumes more energy and produces more waste products than any other system in the body. In fact, you could argue that everything else, organs, blood, nerves, skin, is there to protect, nourish, repair and generally service its every need.

In a healthy body, all these systems interact, working together in harmony. When this balance is disrupted, due to stress or injury, the osteopath's job is to diagnose and treat any faults or breakdowns in the musculo-skeletal framework.

In this sense, osteopathy is a holistic approach, taking into account your way of life, and your mental and emotional state, as important factors influencing total body health. A practitioner will be as concerned about *why* a problem has arisen as with the problem itself. Is your bad back due to a lifetime of lifting heavy loads the wrong way? Could your spine be crooked because an old scar in the abdominal muscles is pulling your body to one side? Does your neck ache because your muscles are taut from years of anxiety and self-doubt? The osteopath can ease the tension with massage, but he will also refer you to a counsellor to deal with the emotional causes.

Osteopaths work with their hands, both for diagnosis and treatment. Years of training and experience have sensitised their fingers, so that by feeling (palpating) the tissues, muscles and joints, and by testing temperature, tone, shape and response to movement, they can detect problem areas.

Osteopathy was founded in the United States in 1874 by Dr Andrew Taylor Still. He believed that when the body was correctly adjusted, there would be less strain on the muscles and joints, all the systems would function smoothly, and the body could heal itself naturally.

It has been a long and, finally, successful struggle for respectability. Popularity came first. In 1991 a *Which?* survey found osteopathy to be the most widely used complementary therapy in Britain. Eight out of ten people said they would use it again, and an estimated 100,000 people go for treatment every week, mainly for back pain. In a more recent survey, patients reported a marked improvement after osteopathy, especially if they sought treatment early on.

In July 1993, the Osteopathy Act was passed, making osteopathy the first non-conventional therapy in the UK to be regulated by law, and putting it on a legal footing with other health professions, such as nursing, dentistry and physiotherapy. Most osteopaths undergo a four-year degree course and some schools now offer graduates the chance to study for an MSc in Osteopathy.

Best for

Back pain, joint pain and strain, arthritis, sciatica, frozen shoulder, cervical spondylosis, rheumatic conditions, sports injuries, pre-menstrual syndrome, asthma. In pregnant women, it can relieve discomfort. In children, certain osteopathic techniques have been used to treat colic, sleeplessness and glue ear. (See also *Cranial osteopathy*.)

What happens

At the first consultation, which may last up to an hour, you will be asked in detail about your medical history and general health, and any drugs or medication you are taking, including homeopathic and herbal remedies The osteopath will want to know about your work, leisure activities, family and emotional state of health.

You will probably be asked to undress to your underwear, so that the practitioner can see as much of your body framework as possible. Women may be offered a gown if they feel uncomfortable. You will be asked to stand, sit and lie down on a treatment table, while the osteopath studies the way you hold yourself and move, and feels (palpates) your tissues, and, perhaps, asks you to bend this way and that while feeling your spine. The osteopath will also test your reflexes and muscle strength together with other standard medical tests. If necessary, arrangements will be made for X-rays and blood tests.

At the end of this, the osteopath will make a diagnosis and decide whether osteopathy can help you, or whether you should be referred to another specialist. For the treatment, you will be asked to lie on a special table. Treatment usually includes massage-type techniques, to relax your muscles; rhythmic movements and stretching, to improve joint mobility; and something called a high velocity thrust. This can cause a joint to 'click', and is sometimes taken for what can seem a 'miracle cure'. The pain accompanying muscle spasm disappears almost by magic, and movement is suddenly possible.

Treatment is rarely painful, and usually rather agreeable, even though you can find yourself in some peculiar positions. One visit may be enough, although the average is anywhere from three to six, depending on your problem. Long-term conditions might need more sessions.

Mike, a 45-year-old bookshop owner, said:

'About five years ago I really put my back out. I was bending down to pick something up and just moved the wrong way, and suddenly I was in screaming agony. I was treated with painkillers, physiotherapy and massage, but that just seemed to be playing around, dulling the pain but nothing else. There was an osteopath at the local complementary health centre who was recommended, so I went to see him. He had a good look at me, told me to hop up on the table, and gave my back an almighty crack. Wham! It wasn't violent, but very strong, and I walked away feeling completely different.

'I play a lot of tennis and lift a lot of heavy boxes of books in my job, and now I make an appointment with him whenever I feel my back's been under strain, and go out feeling as if I'm walking on air. He's also very keen on stretching exercises, almost like yoga, and these are a great help too.'

Most osteopaths are in private practice (check your health insurance if you have it; you may be covered). Expect to pay £20 to £30 for the first visit and £15 to £30 for subsequent visits, which usually last half an hour. You may be able to get osteopathy on the NHS, as some GPs now have contracts for osteopathic treatment. The BMA have called upon the General Medical Council to allow doctors to refer patients to practitioners such as osteopaths

who are statutorily recognised. In practice, many GPs find their
budget will not stretch to it, which is unfortunate because a few
sessions of osteopathy could well save hours of expensive treatment
and NHS drugs.

Doctors say

Despite evidence that osteopathy is an effective treatment, especially
for back pain, some doctors are still suspicious. The profession's
new legal status should attract funds for research that will convince
even the most entrenched sceptics.

Rating

Popularity	Medical Credibility	Scientific Research	Availability
✰✰✰✰	✰✰✰✰	✰✰✰✰	✰✰✰✰

POLARITY THERAPY

According to this therapy, ill health is due to blockages in the body's
energy currents – energy here being a Western variation of Chinese
Qi and Ayurvedic *prana*. The therapy was developed in the US by
Dr Randolph Stone (1890–1983), an Austrian-born naturopath,
chiropractor and osteopath, who studied yoga and Eastern
medicine.

Energy, it is claimed, moves between positive and negative poles in
different parts of the body (feet and palm of the left hand are said to
negative, while the head and right palm are positive), passing through
five energy centres which are neutral and correspond to the Eastern
chakras. These are known as ether, air, fire, water and earth.

Polarity practitioners believe that blockages in this flow are caused
by poor diet and eating habits, emotional and psychological problems
and stress. They attempt to rebalance energy by means of manipulation and touch, stretching postures, attention to diet, and the
encouragement of a better mental attitude.

Best for

Polarity therapy would claim to relieve any condition as the aim
is to achieve balance in the body, although specific symptoms are
claimed to be relieved by treating underlying energy blocks.

What happens

The practitioner takes your medical history and asks about your
general health and lifestyle, before analysing the subtle energy
anatomy, devised by Dr Stone, which underlies the body's systems.
This diagnosis is carried out alongside treatment.

Through touch and manipulation, the practitioner's hands are used
to release blockages in this energy and then balance or 'polarise' it
between the positive and negative poles. Pressure varies in intensity,
from neutral, a light soothing fingertip touch to ease balance; to
positive, which aims to move energy by manipulating various
parts of the body; and negative, a strong and sometimes painful
manipulation of deep body tissues to disperse blockages.

Stretching postures, which vary from the gentle to the active, are
accompanied by vocalisation. These are designed to open up
energy flow, tone the muscles, release toxins and strengthen the
spine. Several diets are recommended; one is the 'cleansing' diet,
a regime of 'live' foods such as fresh fruit and vegetables and a
detoxifying drink called 'liverflush', a mixture of lemon juice,
olive oil, garlic and ginger root. Another is the 'health-building'
diet, that gradually reintroduces foods into what will become
a vegetarian diet.

Counselling explores negative attitudes towards life. and positive
approaches are encouraged to stimulate mental energy. Sessions
last one hour and cost £15 to £30.

Doctors say

The theory of energy flow is based on Oriental philosophy, and
no scientific evidence for it exists to satisfy Western medicine.
However, there is little harm in the treatments (though it would be
wise to check with your GP before embarking on a detoxifying diet)
and possibly some good, provided your doctor has diagnosed any
symptoms.

Rating

Popularity	Medical Credibility	Scientific Research	Availability
★★	★★	★★	★★★

PSYCHOTHERAPY

'I can't cope.' 'Things are really getting me down.' Everyone feels like this at times, especially as the pace of modern life whirls along faster and faster. Stress, anxiety, grief, depression, phobias – all can become overwhelming, but to whom and where can you turn for help? Those who traditionally offered emotional support – priests, family doctors, wise old relatives and neighbours – are in short supply in modern society, where families are scattered hundreds of miles apart, churchgoing is no longer the norm, and the GP can spare ten minutes if you are lucky.

Some problems are too intimate or shocking to discuss with friends, who know you too well to be detached. On such occasions, it can be a relief to pour out everything to an understanding and objective stranger, someone who is trained to listen attentively and help you find your own answers. 'A therapist is trained to spot the important things which are *not* said,' said a psychotherapist, 'and should have the knowledge to make links between present behaviour and things in the past.'

More people than ever, literally hundreds of thousands in the UK, are turning to counsellors and psychotherapists. A growing number of GP practices employ counsellors, and many doctors prefer to recommend therapy that might resolve a problem, rather than prescribe drugs that will only push it into the background. In business and industry, enlightened companies that recognise the link between personal problems and work performance are providing counselling services for employees.

When should you seek help?

Life's rough patches are usually due to one or more of what practitioners call the 'Three Cs'.

Choice You are paralysed because you cannot decide what step to take next. Should you get married? Switch to a new career? The indecision and muddle is affecting your work and relationships.

Change Bereavement, divorce, parenthood, midlife, retirement – these are major life events when you move from one phase to another, and the strength of the feelings that are stirred up can take you by surprise.

Confusion You may be distressed and cannot understand why; either the causes are too deep-seated to break into consciousness, or you know the reason, but you cannot prevent the emotional aftermath that is blighting your life. Your marriage may be unhappy; your job is getting you down; or you are unreasonably anxious about your children and parents.

Provided you find the right therapy and the right practitioner, the experience can be enormously beneficial and, in some cases, life-changing. In a survey reported by Which?, two thirds of those people who had therapy improved.

Who does what

Psychotherapy and counselling are the two professions most likely to be considered complementary, but it is useful to know what the other 'psychs' do.

Psychiatrists train as doctors and then specialise in mental problems. They tend to treat patients primarily with drugs, although some offer psychotherapy. They have not necessarily been in personal therapy themselves.

Psychologists take a science-based university degree, studying the mind and behaviour. They may then specialise as educational, occupational, experimental, social or clinical psychologists. The latter deal with emotional and behavioural problems, working in many areas of the NHS, and using a variety of psychotherapeutic methods, usually behavioural and cognitive (see below).

Psychoanalysts attempt to explain behaviour as the interplay between the conscious and unconscious mind. This 'talking cure' was pioneered by Sigmund Freud, who believed that unacceptable primitive instincts were banished to the unconscious, and surfaced in dreams, creative actitivies and psychiatric illness. Traditionally depicted as sitting behind a couch while the 'patient' dredges up childhood traumas, psychoanalysts often insist that clients attend three to five 50-minute sessions a week for several years. The technique has evolved, particularly under the influence of Carl Jung, and psychoanalysis is now considered as one of several kinds of psychotherapy.

Psychotherapists help you examine your past experiences and relationships in order to deal with deep-seated personal issues that can bring about profound changes in the way you think and behave. One practitioner compared it with disentangling a knot: 'You loosen one bit, and some of it unravels, and then you work at another piece until that is freed, and finally everything is released.'

A crucial element in this therapy is *transference*, in which your emotional response to an important figure in your life is transferred to the practitioner. You might react to the practitioner's questions, for example, in the same defensive way you did with, say, your father. Both psychotherapists and psychoanalysts have been in therapy themselves as part of their training.

Treatment tends to be long term; weekly visits for six months would be the minimum, and two years or more the norm.

Counsellors tend to focus on a specific problem, such as bereavement, and the treatment is viewed in terms of weeks, rather than months or years. He or she will be supportive, skilled in listening and prompting, but will give little or no direct advice. The aim is to help you draw on your own resources to gain insight into your problems. You will be encouraged to stand up for yourself if depressed or lacking in confidence, or enabled to express difficult emotions such as anger or fear. Training is shorter and less academic than that of the other professionals, and a good counsellor knows when to refer a client for more expert treatment.

In practice, *counselling* and *psychotherapy* can overlap and this adds to the confusion. 'Psychodynamic counsellors' offer what others might call psychotherapy. The psychotherapist you see in private practice could be called a counsellor when working at the student health centre.

Which therapy?

Psychotherapists and counsellors use an overwhelming number of therapies, and trying to sort out which might be right for you is a daunting task. Even those in the business find it next to impossible. Try to be as clear as possible in advance about what kind of therapy you seek. Do you want it to be 'warm' (i.e. friendly and supportive), or 'cool' (analytic and detached)? Do you want to work on your feelings or on your thinking and behaviour? Would you prefer the practitioner to be in charge, or do you need to be in control? Do you like more of an equal relationship? Or would you feel more comfortable working in a group of people rather than one to one?

Therapies you are likely to encounter include:

Behavioural therapy This is based on the idea that our behaviour is learnt in response to our environment, and can be changed when we meet different circumstances. It means that we can unlearn problem behaviour, and replace it with something better without spending hours digging into past traumas. Various mental and physical exercises, including punishment and reward strategies, are employed to lever you out of your rut. It works very well with stress-related illness and irrational fears and phobias. For example, someone with a crippling fear of flying is taught relaxation, given information about aerodynamics and taken to the airport to look at planes.

Cognitive therapy Previous experiences condition you to think about yourself in a particular way, which in turn affects your attitudes and emotions, and the way that you deal with situations. By changing your thinking, you will change your behaviour. Someone with a poor self-image and lack of confidence, for example, will be taught to replace negative opinons of self with upbeat positive ones.

Gestalt therapy Developed by German psychoanalyst, Fritz Perls, in California in the 1960s, this therapy aims to make people aware of their thoughts and actions by making them conscious of their immediate behaviour, particularly their non-verbal body language. One of the techniques used is 'talking to the empty chair', in which you imagine that part of yourself – an emotion, a person in your life, part of your body – is sitting opposite you and you can address them freely. The process, which is usually conducted in two- or three-day workshop groups, generates startling and profoundly expressive responses. It is said to be particularly effective for those who are tense and anxious or have difficulties communicating their feelings to others.

Group therapy People meet in small groups, usually of no more than ten, to share personal experiences and feelings. A unique bond can develop between members as groups meet over a number of weeks and months. This therapy is helpful for those with emotional difficulties and problems in dealing with people, and is a very supportive way of treating addiction.

Humanistic psychotherapy This approach embraces a number of practices (including Gestalt therapy), many of them springing from the 'personal growth movement' of the 1960s, and owing much to American psychotherapists Carl Rogers and Abraham Maslow. The emphasis is on your inner life and your feelings about yourself and your circumstances. By exploring these, you are encouraged to take responsibility for your thoughts and actions, aiming for 'high-level wellness' rather than unravelling neuroses.

Neurolinguistic programming (NLP) One of the newer therapies that suddenly seem to be everywhere, it is based on the assumption that our personal experiences colour the way we perceive the world. When we discover how this happens, it is said we can take control of the process, sometimes by changing the way we speak and move, so that we communicate better, learn more rapidly, and bring about behaviour changes in ourselves and others.

Psychodrama Groups of people take turns to act out each other's real-life situations and problems. Explosive emotions can be released, both for actors and observers, which the practitioner may use to help people accept their feelings and learn new ways of dealing with problems. It can be very effective for people who find it hard to relate to friends or family, or who feel inhibited.

Psychosynthesis Based on the principles of Italian psychiatrist, Roberto Assagioli, this aims at developing a balanced personality and exploring higher levels of consciousness in order to achieve your maximum potential, in all aspects of your life. Through painting, imagery, movement and diary-writing, you gain knowledge of the different facets of your personality and learn to realise your true creative self. It is an inspiring method of personal growth, and therapeutic for those suffering from stress and relationship problems or a 'crisis of meaning'.

Transactional Analysis (TA) Developed by Canadian psychiatrist, Eric Berne, who wrote the best-selling *Games People Play* in 1964. Everyone carries a child, an adult and a parent self within him or her, and every situation in which we engage with other people evokes one of these selves. For example, a tired woman coming home late from work might hope her partner will play the parent and cook supper for the child in her. Through learning about these strategies or 'transactions', people (it is hoped) will understand their own behaviour and be able to choose which role to play.

(See also *Art therapy*, *Dance movement therapy*, *Hypnotherapy*, *Music therapy*, *Sound therapy* and *Voice therapy*.)

What happens
Each therapy has its own particular approach, so it is difficult to generalise. The first interview is an opportunity for you and the practitioner to get to know each other (many will agree to a free consultation – they are also deciding whether they can help *you*), and you are entitled to ask some searching questions:

- What qualifications does the practitioner have, and what was the training?

- How many years has the practitioner been in practice?

- Is the practitioner a member of a professional organisation?

- Does the practitioner receive regular supervision from another practitioner (every qualified practitioner needs this)?

- What is the practitioner's approach? What can you expect to happen during the sessions?

- How long is the course of therapy likely to last? (At an *average* fee of £30 for a 50-minute session it could prove expensive.)

- Will there be regular reviews of the way the therapy is progressing?

If therapy is going to be helpful, you must feel comfortable about revealing a great deal of your innermost thoughts and feelings to the practitioner; if you have any doubts at all, or if at any time you are uneasy about anything suggested, then discuss it, and remember you can always stop the therapy.

Jo, a 34-year-old marketing consultant, told of her experience:

'My marriage was very shaky, and I was having problems working with a colleague at the office. I felt really miserable and couldn't see how to improve things. A friend suggested I see a psychotherapist and recommended David.

'I didn't know what to expect. At the first consultation we both kind of sussed each other out. He asked me general questions about my problems and background, and then said he would take me on if I was still interested, but I must commit myself to coming each week for three months, and we would then review the situation.

'He's a psychoanalytical psychotherapist, and very careful to not let slip anything about himself that might hinder what they call transference, placing feelings I might have about other people on to him. Although he sees clients at home, you enter his study directly through a side door so you don't get any impression of his private life.

'You arrive, and sit down on a sofa with a box of tissues on a sidetable, and he's opposite in an easy chair, and then he just waits for you to start. Sooner or later you say something to fill the gap, and then it all seems to come spilling out. I found that I needed to talk, absolutely endlessly and compulsively, about myself, all kinds of silly, horrible things that you'd never tell a friend. When I burst into tears, which was rather often, David didn't say anything but just handed me the tissues. Occasionally he asks the odd question to keep me going, or makes a statement that rounds things up.

'I was fascinated at how, once I started exploring my early childhood and the feelings that came up about my parents, things began to fall into place. You understand what's behind your reactions to people and events now, and that seems to help you see what to do. The trouble I had dealing with the woman at work had a lot to do with my relationship with my mother.

'After three months, I decided to continue. I've been seeing David for just over a year now, and I feel I've gone as far as I want for the moment, so we're working towards stopping in three weeks time. My marriage is better, and I'm happier in my job.'

Doctors say

Most doctors are sympathetic to psychotherapy and counselling, and would agree that the right kind of therapy can be enormously beneficial, provided you see a qualified practitioner. Some methods can trigger repressed and traumatic emotions that you may not be ready to confront, and if this happens you will need experienced counselling.

Rating

Popularity	Medical Credibility	Scientific Research	Availability
★★★★	★★★★	★★★★	★★★★

QI GONG

Relatively unheard of five years ago and increasingly popular, qi gong (translatable as 'energy cultivation') is an ancient Chinese system of exercises in posture, breathing and focusing the mind, that aims to develop and strengthen your internal energy, and control the circulation of the life force known as Qi. There are many types of qi gong (it has been compared to the different varieties of music, from classical to rock), but they can be largely divided into static and moving, hard and soft. T'ai chi ch'uan, for example, is a form of qi gong.

Rating

Popularity	Medical Credibility	Scientific Research	Availability
✰✰	✰	✰	✰

RADIONICS AND RADIESTHESIA

Dowsing is the ability of the human body to pick up 'good' or 'bad' vibrations from hidden energy sources, a principle that was applied to disease in the 1920s by a French priest, Abbé Mermet, who used a pendulum to 'dowse' patients in the local hospital. Radiesthesia, meaning 'sensitivity to radiation', was the name he gave to this kind of medical diagnosis.

Radionics works on the same principles, but uses instruments to diagnose and heal at a distance – although practitioners prefer the word 'analyse'. Their intention is not to diagnose and name a disease, they say, but to put together a holistic picture of your physical, mental and emotional health. In this way, disharmonies and distortions in our individual energy patterns can be identified and measured.

At much the same time that Abbé Mermet was dowsing in France, an American neurologist, Albert Abrams, discovered that the sound made by tapping (percussing) the body of a patient varied according to the area percussed and the nature of the disease. In addition, Abrams invented a 'black box' that could, without any electronic circuitry or power source, allegedly pick up abnormal radiations (or 'bioenergy') from a piece of diseased tissue – a 'witness', such as a hair, or drop of blood. The patient need not be present at all.

His medical colleagues were sceptical, and many purchasers of the box complained that they got no response from it. After his death in 1924, an American chiropractor, Ruth Drown, developed his work, but she was prosecuted by the US Food and Drug Administration (FDA), and convicted of fraud and quackery.

In Britain, engineer, George De La Warr, formed the Radionic and Magnetic Centre in 1965, and not only produced instruments that claimed to measure bioenergy but a 'camera' that, when a spot of blood was inserted into it, produced photographs of the internal organs. As his boxes failed to work in test conditions, he, too, was arrested for fraud, but acquitted, because the jury decided that he genuinely believed in what he was selling.

What happens

You may never meet your radionics practitioner face to face. After making contact, you are sent a questionnaire to fill in, listing past medical history and present symptoms. You return this with your 'witness,' either a drop of your blood on lint or litmus paper, or a lock of your hair.

The practitioner focuses his or her mind on you, and tunes one of the radionic instruments to the energy waves that are said to be emitted by your 'witness'; a series of dials with frequency settings corresponds to various disorders. The practitioner may also 'dowse' the written list of symptoms on your questionnaire with a pendulum, and, once an analysis of your condition is made, may broadcast healing waves to you with another radionics instrument, or contact you with suggestions for further treatment with other therapies.

And that is all, until you are sent the bill, which is usually about £38 for the first two-hour analysis, and then £28 per month for treatment.

Doctors say

Given their past experience at the hands of sceptical scientists and the law, radionics practitioners are rather wary of clinical trials and inclined to get on with individual healing practice. In 1924, however, a British medical committee, under the chairmanship of Sir Thomas (later Lord) Horder, conducted a series of controlled experiments with a version of Abrams's black box. To the astonishment of the doctors involved, it appeared to work, but the experiments have never been repeated.

Most doctors today remain highly sceptical of the principles of radionics. The kindest comment some of them would make is that it may be a form of *distant healing,* in which case instruments would not be necessary.

Rating

Popularity	Medical Credibility	Scientific Research	Availability
✮✮	✮	✮	✮✮

REFLEXOLOGY

Could pressure on your big toe relieve your headache? According to reflexologists, every part of the body is reflected (hence the term 'reflexology') in our feet. By pressing and massaging the soles and toes, energy is unblocked and our natural healing powers enhanced to restore balance.

Imagine that the sole of the foot is the body, the big toe the head, the waist a line crossing at the instep. The lungs are somewhere around the ball of the foot, and the small intestine and bladder are towards the heel.

Reflexologists say that ten vertical energy lines, or 'zones', run from the feet, up the body to the head, and down to the hands, also used in treatment. Organs and structures within each zone are connected by a flow of energy. In theory, any accessible point in the zone can be used to treat another, but the feet are preferred, because they are more sensitive.

Despite the obvious similarity to the *meridians* (energy channels) of *Traditional Chinese Medicine*, most practitioners insist that it is a separate system.

Foot massage is not new – an ancient Egyptian tomb painting shows two men manipulating the feet and hands of two others – but it was an American ear, nose and throat specialist, Dr William H. Fitzgerald, who introduced the concept of *zone therapy* in 1915. Another American, physiotherapist Eunice Ingham, took it further, maintaining that all parts of the body could be treated by pressing relevant areas of the feet. One of her students, Doreen Bayly, introduced reflexology to the UK in the 1960s, and its popularity has rocketed since. It is relatively easy to learn, simple to perform, and, in theory, anyone can do it.

Best for

Apart from relaxation and the identification of possible problem areas (the reflexologist will advise you to see a doctor if it is considered there is an undiagnosed ailment), it is claimed that more than a hundred medical conditions can benefit from this form of therapy, including acne, some allergies, eczema, psoriasis, gastrointestinal disorders (heartburn, constipation, diarrhoea), stress-related problems such as asthma and migraine, menstrual problems and pain.

What happens

Treatment lasts about 45 to 60 minutes, and can take place at home or in a centre. You will be asked questions about past and present health, and something about your lifestyle, before settling back in a reclining chair with your bare feet raised. The practitioner then examines your feet, applying pressure to all areas with the hands and thumbs. A feeling of sharpness or tenderness points to crystalline deposits beneath the skin, an indication that an area of the body is out of balance – the greater the reaction, the greater the imbalance. All areas of the feet are massaged, so that the body as a whole is treated, and extra massage is given to tender areas.

A number of treatments may be required, with at least a week between appointments. Expect to pay £14 to £30, depending on where you live. Reflexologists say that as the body tries to remove toxins from the system, there may be a 'healing crisis', such as a cough, runny nose or rash.

Jane, a 39-year-old voluntary worker with two children, said:

'Nothing seemed to clear up my urinary infection, not even antibiotics, and a friend suggested I see a reflexologist. The first visit was very painful, when she worked on specific areas of my foot, and within hours of getting home I had a temperature of 102 degrees, and all my symptoms were back with a vengeance. When I rang the reflexologist, she said 'good'. Apparently my body was getting rid of toxins, and the reaction had disappeared in the morning.

'I went about six times, and, unlike other occasions when I've had reflexology for relaxation, these therapeutic sessions left me

absolutely shattered and feeling rather awful. But the infection cleared up – although I suppose it could also have been the antibiotics eventually taking effect.'

Doctors say

In one of the few clinical trials in reflexology, a Californian study found that 83 per cent of women who had weekly reflexology massage reported that premenstrual symptoms were reduced by as much as 30 per cent, compared with 24 per cent of a group given a placebo massage. The theory of zones and energy lines is unsubstantiated by anything in current scientific knowledge, however, and some of the benefits reported could be due to the relaxing effects of massage and touch. However, so long as any symptoms of ill-health are reported to your doctor, you can relax and enjoy it!

Rating

Popularity	Medical Credibility	Scientific Research	Availability
☆☆☆☆	☆☆☆	☆☆	☆☆☆☆

RELAXATION AND BREATHING

Relaxation and breathing should be the most natural things in the world, but it is surprising how many people find the first impossible and do the second wrongly. Being able to relax at will is the best possible way of dealing with stress; it lowers the blood pressure, breathing and metabolic rate, and slows the heartbeat, enabling the body's systems to recover from over-arousal.

When under stress, we also tend to breathe in a quick, shallow way from the top of our chest, but, if we do this all the time, we are actively reinforcing body messages of stress and fear to our already overloaded brain. Abdominal or diaphragmatic breathing uses the diaphragm, the sheet of muscle between the chest cavity and the abdomen, to allow efficient, relaxed expansion of the lungs: it is relaxation breathing as in sleep breathing. This ensures adequate supplies of oxygen to the body without expelling too much carbon dioxide – a substance the blood needs in just the right amount to maintain its optimum level of acidity.

Check that you are breathing from the diaphragm by lying on your back and putting one hand on your chest and the other on your abdomen. Notice which hand is moving when you breathe in and out. If it is the hand on your chest, then you're breathing incorrectly. Concentrate on pulling in your the stomach muscles as you breathe out, pushing them in gently if necessary with your hand, to train yourself to breathe deeply from the diaphragm.

Relaxation can take a bit of practice, especially if you are inclined to be tense, but once achieved, the sensation becomes easier to recognise and sink into again.

Try the following for deep muscle relaxation

- Choose a time when you have not just finished a heavy meal.

- Make sure your clothes are loose and comfortable and your feet covered for warmth.

- Ensure the room is warm and that you will not be disturbed for at least 15 minutes.

- Lie flat on your back on a firm bed, or on a rug or mat on the floor. Put a cushion under your head and/or knees if you feel uncomfortable. Your head, body and legs should be in a straight line, your feet flopped loosely, and your hands resting by your side, palms upwards.

- Close your eyes and take a couple of deep, sighing breaths through your nose, taking the breath down to the diaphragm.

- Focus your mind on each part of the body in turn for a few seconds, imagining it relaxing, softening and melting into the floor. Start at your right toes, heel, ankle, leg, knee, thigh and hip. Repeat from your left toes. Then right fingers, hand, wrist, forearm, elbow, upper arm, shoulder. Repeat on the left side. Then from the base of the spine, lower back to upper back. Relax your chest and abdomen. Then neck, jaw, lips, tongue, cheeks, eye muscles, forehead and scalp.

- You should feel so totally relaxed that movement seems impossible. Breathe in and out gently. On each outward breath tell yourself you are more relaxed, more peaceful …

- Stay like this for at least five, and preferably ten, minutes.

- Open your eyes, take a deep breath, stir your limbs gently, then stretch, turn on your side, and get up.

- Practise this at least once a day. Twice if possible.

Rating

Popularity	Medical Credibility	Scientific Research	Availability
✫✫✫✫	✫✫✫✫	✫✫✫✫	✫✫✫✫

ROLFING

In rolfing, the body is compared to a child's tower of bricks; if any of the blocks is out of alignment, then the structure is unstable; too far out, and it would collapse. But, being human, our mind and muscles work twice as hard to keep us standing up and moving about. This constant effort, it is said, can leave us drained of vitality and prone to illness.

Life events and stresses are blamed for distorting the body in the first place, and poor posture continues to affect our feelings, so that people can be described as 'tense with rage' or 'bowed with grief'.

Rolfing or 'structural integration', developed by American biological chemist, Dr Ida Rolf (1896–1979), is a system of deep massage and manipulation of the connective tissue and muscles that aims to release the pain that may be crippling us, loosen up the body and realign it in a straight vertical line. Only then, it is claimed, can the earth's gravity field, support the body's energy field and our natural powers of self-healing work unimpeded.

119

Best for

Those who feel they would profit from it and are interested in personal growth. Rolfing is not designed to treat specific disorders, nor is it recommended in cases of organic disease.

What happens

Treatment usually consists of ten weekly, one-hour sessions, at about £50 per session. Each is devoted to a particular body area, even the inside of the mouth. You undress as far as your underpants, and the practitioner photographs you from the front, back and sides to detect any abnormal body posture. Then you lie on a massage couch or on the floor, and the practitioner manipulates your muscles and connective tissue with knuckles, elbows, hands and fingers, using his or her own weight to apply pressure. This is not a soothing process; in fact it is often uncomfortable and even painful, both physically and emotionally. Some people end up half an inch taller as a result.

Doctors say

So long as you are not trying to treat a particular disorder, feel confident about your practitioner and regard it as a means of personal growth, then choosing this form of therapy is up to you.

Rating

Popularity	Medical Credibility	Scientific Research	Availability
✫✫✫	✫✫✫	✫✫✫	✫✫

SHAMANISM

The current popularity of Native American traditions has aroused an interest in Shamanism. In tribal societies, from the ancient Celts to Australian aborigines, the shaman – a kind of wizard, witchdoctor, wise man or woman, priest or priestess, according to the nature of the culture – was believed to have special mental, spiritual and even physical powers, and to be able to communicate with the supernatural world. The advice of the shaman was sought for diagnosis and treatment of all kinds of physical and psychological conditions.

Shamanism today emphasises the importance of balance and harmony in the natural world, and the practice of the 'way of the four directions'. This involves honouring the four kingdoms of animal, plant, mineral and human; the four elements of earth, air, fire and water; the four aspects of humanity – physical, mental, emotional and spiritual.

Rating

Popularity	Medical Credibility	Scientific Research	Availability
☆	☆	☆	☆

SHIATSU

Shiatsu has been said to combine some of the best elements of Western and Oriental medicine in one technique. The word is Japanese for 'finger pressure', and the therapy is a combination of massage, pressure on the *acupoints* (key spots on the *meridians* – energy channels that, according to *Traditional Chinese Medicine*, run through the body) and components of physiotherapy and chiropractic.

Chinese massage blended well with a Japanese variation called *anma* when Chinese medicine was adopted by the Japanese about 1500 years ago. Over the centuries, however, the healing element was forgotten and anma became simply a means of relaxation and pleasure. It was reinstated as a serious therapy early in the twentieth century, under the new name of 'shiatsu.'

The shiatsu practitioner uses the fingers, thumbs, elbows, knees, and even feet to exert pressure on the acupoints (known in Japanese as tsubo), where the universal life energy Qi (ki in Japanese) is said to enter and exit the body and is most intensely concentrated. Stimulating these points can free the flow of Qi where it is blocked, and restore it to depleted areas, thus maintaining healthy harmony.

The Shiatsu Society translates this into Western physiology as stimulating blood circulation and the flow of lymphatic fluid, helping to release toxins and tension from the muscles, and stimulating the hormonal system. On a more subtle level, it adds, shiatsu allows you to relax deeply and get in touch with your body's healing abilities. Treatment should leave a feeling of calm and well-being.

Best for

Shiatsu is a health-promoting therapy, so anyone can benefit from treatment, but it is claimed to be especially helpful for stress-related conditions, such as headaches and migraine, tension, anxiety and depression, insomnia, fatigue and weakness; asthma, bronchitis, sinus trouble, catarrh, digestive disorders and bowel trouble, painful menstruation and some other uro-genital conditions, circulatory problems (though not with haemorrhage or thrombosis), rheumatic and arthritic complaints, back trouble, sciatica and conditions following sprains and injuries. Care should be taken in pregnancy, or where there is tissue or bone damage, or a suspected tumour.

What happens

Like other complementary practitioners, Shiatsu practitioners are interested in the whole person, rather than in focusing on the symptoms or the disease. They are trained in the four methods of Chinese diagnosis, and so they will ask you detailed questions about your past and present health and lifestyle; *observe* your posture, the way you walk and sit, your hair, your face – are the puffy bags under your eyes a sign of disrupted kidney energy? They will *listen* to your voice: is it whiny (dysfunctional lung energy) or sharp (possible problems in the liver energy)? And they will pay attention to any intuitive reactions they may receive about you. Finally, they will diagnose by *touch*, including the Japanese abdominal or 'Hara' diagnosis, feeling the abdomen to determine how the energy flows in the internal organs.

For treatment you remain clothed, but wear something loose, preferably cotton, like a track or jogging suit. To gain the most benefit, you are advised to avoid alcohol on the day of treatment, eat lightly, and not to take a long, hot bath – shower if you can.

You lie down on a mat (usually a futon) on the floor, as this makes it easier for the practitioner to apply pressure. Treatment is given in four ways: pressing the body at right angles, sometimes with the knee or elbow, to increase the flow of blood and energy; stretching and squeezing to break up energy blockages; rocking to counteract agitations in the energy flow; and gentle holding on the meridians or specific points to enhance the flow of energy.

At the end you will be left alone for a few minutes to relax and let the benefits sink in. Sometimes there can be after effects – flu-like symptoms, aches and pains – that are known as a 'healing crisis', said to be a sign that the body is trying to expel toxins released as energy is unblocked.

Sessions usually last about one hour, and you can expect to pay £20 to £30. Several treatments may be necessary, depending on your particular condition.

Doctors say

As with acupressure, a stimulating massage helps produce endorphins, the body's pain-relieving hormones. Shiatsu will not interfere with any other treatment you might be having, provided you tell the practitioner of any medication or known health problems, such as cancer or heart disease, and report any symptoms of ill-health to your GP.

Rating

Popularity	Medical Credibility	Scientific Research	Availability
✰✰✰	✰✰	✰✰	✰✰✰

SOUND THERAPY

Sound waves vibrate at different frequencies of energy. Those that we can hear are in the middle range, but there are frequencies too high for the human ear (ultrasonics) and too low (infrasonics). Relentless noise such as traffic, pneumatic drills, loud rock music and low-flying aircraft is a notorious cause of stress, just as the cooing of doves, the crooning of a mother to her child or certain musical notes can be soothing (airlines are said to find Bach excellent for calming passengers waiting for take-off). (See also *Music therapy*, *Dance movement therapy* and *Voice therapy*.)

Different body tissues vary in their absorption or reflection of sound waves. Conventional medicine makes use of this fact to target and disintegrate kidney stones and gall stones with high-intensity sound energy (lithotripsy) and, diagnostically, to scan the foetus in the womb. Physiotherapists also use sound waves to break down tissue adhesions that cause muscular pain and inflammation of joints.

In complementary medicine, it is believed that each cell of the body vibrates at a particular frequency. In good health this is constant, but a disrupted rhythm is symptomatic of disease. *Cymatics* practitioners use tape recordings and electronic devices to generate sound waves intended to compress and expand the cells at a rate that will restore them to their proper harmony.

Best for
Muscle and bone problems such as rheumatoid arthritis, fibrositis, sprains and myalgia are said to respond to this therapy.

Doctors say
Apart from the demonstrable uses of sound waves in orthodox medicine, there is no evidence that sound can affect cellular vibrations in a therapeutic way.

Rating

Popularity	Medical Credibility	Scientific Research	Availability
☆☆	☆☆	☆☆	☆☆

T'AI CHI CH'UAN

'Meditation in motion' is the description most often applied to the slow, graceful, circular movements of this exercise. The origins are rather lost in the mists of time, but it is believed to have been developed by an eleventh century Chinese thinker, Chang San-Feng, who blended Taoist philosophy with martial arts movements (*ch'uan* is Chinese for 'fist', *t'ai chi* means 'wholeness' or 'ultimate').

By focusing not only the body but the mind and emotions on the performance of a series of postures, known by such beautiful, symbolic names as 'snake creeps down to water' and 'the stork cools its wings', the life energy of the body (called Qi in *Traditional Chinese Medicine*), is encouraged to flow evenly.

When our Qi is out of balance because it is blocked, or concentrated in one area of the body and depleted in another, natural harmony is said to be disrupted and we are susceptible to illnesses. T'ai chi ch'uan is a method for tuning ourselves up physically, mentally and spiritually, the aim being to become at one with Qi.

Ideally, it should be practised in the open air, where the earth forces of universal Qi can be drawn up and expressed through the hands – which is why visitors to China see so many serene people performing T'ai-chi in parks, and even in the streets.

Best for
General mental and physical control and stress-related conditions such as anxiety and tension.

What happens
Ideally, you need instruction from a qualified teacher, one who has at least four years experience. The 'forms' are a series of postures linked in one long flowing movement. The 'short form' consists of 37 movements that can be performed in five or ten minutes; the 'long form' takes 20 to 40 minutes, and has 108 movements.

Classes should be quiet and calm, with an unhurried atmosphere, and the teacher should explain the philosophy behind the movements.

Doctors say

Some cardiologists are said to have prescribed T'ai chi for heart patients, to lower blood pressure and calm hostility. Certainly there is nothing to harm you in this exercise, and every likelihood of doing some good.

Rating

Popularity	Medical Credibility	Scientific Research	Availability
✰✰✰	✰✰	✰	✰✰✰✰

THERAPEUTIC TOUCH

This appears in practice to be similar to spiritual healing, or the 'laying on of hands,' but health professionals who use the therapy explain it in terms of a branch of physics, known as quantum mechanics.

According to practitioners, all human beings are energy fields, part of a universal life force. This energy extends beyond the body and interacts with the environment. Ill-health results from imbalances or blockages in this force flow, which the practitioner tries to repattern – sometimes without physical contact with the patient – so that the body's natural healing powers are released. If this still sounds uncannily like spiritual healing, advocates insist there are profound and subtle differences.

'Therapeutic Touch is built on quantum mechanics, the division of modern physics that sees the universe as a dynamic web of correlated events,' declared Jean Sayre-Adams, an American nurse and founder and director of the Didsbury Trust, a charity dedicated to the education and support of health care professionals through the healing arts.

At least 30,000 American nurses practise Therapeutic Touch in hospitals and clinics in the US, and Ms Sayre-Adams has trained several hundred British nurses in administering the therapy.

Hospital authorities are sceptical, however, and few nurses are able to use it – at least officially – in the wards.

Best for

Anxiety, fatigue, headache and other stress-related conditions; sinus, wound healing, pain relief, long muscle pain and emotional and spiritual distress.

What happens

The practitioner sits beside the patient and 'centres' on the present situation, putting personal thoughts aside, mind calm, alert and open, and in harmony with the patient. Without this centreing, the practitioner risks draining her own energy levels.

Then, with the hands the practitioner assesses the nature of the energy field that is the patient. Does it feel warm? Tingly? Buzzy? By sweeping the hands downwards, slightly above the patient's body, areas of imbalance are said to be cleared and the flow restored.

The practitioner concentrates on particularly knotty or blocked areas, using powerful visual images to rebalance energy patterns. One nurse said she pictured a bolt of energy passing down her arm to the patient, who told her later that she felt as if she had been lifted off the floor.

A senior nurse who studied Therapeutic Touch (TT) reported:

'Without actually touching her, I passed my hands over a colleague who was acting as a patient. I felt an area like ice above her pelvis. It turned out she had just had cryosurgery to destroy abnormal cells in her cervix by freezing.'

Another woman, troubled for years with lower back pain, asked a nurse to give her Therapeutic Touch.

'She put her hands on my back and I felt a kind of hot flush. The pain eased, and my back has been a lot better since.'

Doctors say

Although dismissed by the medical establishment, an increasing number of health professionals, doctors and nurses, are interested in the concept of Therapeutic Touch. Those teaching and using it are meticulous about using scientific terminology and avoiding occult or mystical language.

The term was coined in 1972 by Dolores Krieger, Professor of Nursing at New York University, who was exploring ways of harnessing healing power. She later completed experiments that showed the laying on of hands could increase haemoglobin levels in humans.

In further studies, TT proved more effective than casual touch in allaying anxiety. It relieved tension headaches and eased pain in post-operative adults. In complicated experiments, volunteers with minor wounds who received non-contact healing from unseen TT practitioners on the other side of a wall healed faster than the control group.

Rating

Popularity	Medical Credibility	Scientific Research	Availability
✰✰✰	✰✰✰	✰✰✰	✰✰✰

TRADITIONAL CHINESE MEDICINE

This is becoming increasingly popular in the West. *Acupuncture* is probably the best known treatment, but the recent much-publicised success of Chinese herbal medicine in treating eczema, supported by trials at the Great Ormond Street Hospital for Sick Children, has led to long queues to see a particular Chinese doctor in London's Soho. *T'ai chi Ch'uan* and *shiatsu* have also introduced something of the Chinese concept of health to Westerners.

Chinese medicine is not just a question of knowing where to insert needles or which herbs to brew. However, it is very difficult for Western minds to fully grasp the philosophy behind the practice, since it is quite alien to the cause-and-effect approach to which we are conditioned. As a result, some Westerners dismiss talk of yin and yang as hocus-pocus; others go to the opposite extreme, venerating the Chinese system, because it is holistic, as somehow more 'true' and, therefore worthy of reverence.

Neither is the case. As Dr Ted Kaptchuk, a Westerner who spent years training in China, points out, Chinese medicine is an independent system of practice, developed over 4000 years of critical thinking, clinical observation and testing. But, just as it is rooted in the philosophy and habits of a civilisation entirely foreign to our own, so its perceptions of the body, health and disease arise from a very different source. Any explanation of that system in a few pages cannot hope to do it justice. However, a summary could prove useful.

Western doctors start with a symptom, then look for a specific cause, a disease. A Chinese doctor will look at the complete physiological and psychological profile of the individual, of which the symptom is merely one factor, to find 'the pattern of disharmony.' Illness is a result of an imbalance in the flow of qi through the body, and a strong element of Chinese health care – such as T'ai chi – is devoted to preventing such a situation.

Qi (pronounced chee) originally meant air, breath or energy, and then came to mean the vital nourishing and protecting energy. We receive Qi prenatally from our parents, and derive more from food and from air.

Animating Qi is a constant movement of energy between two opposing but complementary forces, *yin* and *yang*. Yin signifies darkness, passivity, coldness, femininity, the negative. Yang signifies light, warmth, action, masculinity, the positive. Each is said to be necessary for the other, and when one predominates, disease and emotional instability can follow.

The yang organs are described as hollow and involved with discharge or absorption, such as the bladder and the stomach. Acute pain, inflammations, spasms, headache and high blood pressure are signs of excess yang.

Yin organs are dense and blood-filled, such as the heart and liver. Excess yin is expressed as dull aches and pains, chilliness, sluggishness, fluid retention and fatigue.

Qi is said to circulate in our body along a network of invisible channels beneath the skin called *meridians*, that run to and from the hands and feet and to the body and head. There are 12 basic meridians, paired on the right and left sides of the body and named after the organs to which they are attached. Six are predominantly yin, six are predominantly yang, and two extra meridians are known as the Conception Vessel and the Governor Vessel.

Dotted along the meridians are the 2000 or so known acupoints, where Qi is said to be concentrated and enters and exits the body. Stimulation of these points, as in acupuncture, acupressure or shiatsu, is claimed to free the flow of Qi, releasing blockages and restoring depletions, thus returning the body to harmony.

Yin and yang can be divided into subcategories of potential disharmony known as the *Eight Principle Patterns*, examples of which would be hot–cold, empty–full. 'Hot' symptoms are a red face and fever; 'cold' would be a slow pulse and pale tongue. If the patient is diagnosed as too hot, the practitioner would try to disperse the heat; if cold, to build up strength.

Another tradition is that of the *Five Elements* or *Five Phases*, qualities described as earth, fire, water, wood and metal, according to which all things in the universe can be organised. Although important in Chinese philosophy, Dr Kaptchuk says that, in reality, Chinese doctors found them too inflexible for medical use, and prefer to work with the concepts of yin and yang. The principles are frequently found in Western explanations of Chinese medicine, however, where they actually seem to work better, possibly because of their stronger mental, emotional and spiritual aspects.

A number of factors can upset the delicate balance of yin and yang: infections, poisons and accidents or trauma; emotional states such as stress, anger or grief; spiritual neglect; inadequate or wrong diet; drugs; weather conditions and genetic inheritance.

Because Chinese medicine regards each individual as a 'whole' entity of body, mind and spirit, a physical disease will affect mental and emotional health, just as an imbalance of emotion will disturb the associated body organ. According to the Nei Jing (the Yellow Emperor's classic text of internal medicine): 'Joy and shock injure the heart, anger injures the liver, worry and overconcentration injure the spleen, grief injures the lungs, fears injure the kidneys.'

Best for

Traditional Chinese medicine is a system in its own right, so would claim to treat any condition.

What happens

You will be assessed according to the 'four methods of diagnosis' – observing, listening and smelling, interrogating, pulse feeling and palpating. The practitioner, for example, will observe the appearance and colour of your face; listen to the sound of your voice; notice any distinctive body odour; ask questions about your medical history, habits such as bowel movements, your work and your family; take your blood pressure, feel your abdomen, and read the six meridian pulses on the left wrist and the six on the right to diagnose illnesses you have suffered, are suffering and may suffer. Your tongue is a whole diagnostic tool in itself – is it red, yellow, mossy, greasy, thick, thin, or dry?

A traditional Chinese doctor will not say: 'You have a peptic ulcer, like thousands of other people, and this is the medicine that we give everybody', but he might say: 'You have a robust constitution, a reddish complexion, and a full, deep voice; you seem assertive and aggressive; you are constipated and your urine is dark and yellow; your tongue has a greasy yellow coating; your pulse is 'full' and 'wiry'. Your pattern of disharmony therefore is called 'Damp Heat Affecting the Spleen."

Once the diagnosis is made, the doctor will determine which treatment is appropriate. This could be acupuncture or moxibustion, which involves burning a herb called moxa, made from the dry leaf of mugwort, in a small cone over an acupuncture point. It might be massage or a herbal infusion.

Chinese herbs are classified into properties such as Hot, Cold, Warm, Cool, and are prescribed accordingly to eliminate imbalances; for example, to calm heat or to expel wind.

Chinese herbal medicine is very fashionable in the UK at present, and *when used correctly* does seem to be effective. However, because the herbs are not classed as medicines, they can be imported and sold without quality checks or evidence of toxicity. Some of them are very toxic indeed; at least 70 women who took a slimming treatment (unheard of in Chinese medicine) that included Chinese herbs are now suffering from severe kidney damage.

Doctors say

When used by qualified practitioners, and in context, Chinese medicine appears to be effective, although most Western doctors cannot accept the concepts of Qi or yin and yang. An electro-magnetic force, which would not be anatomically apparent, has been suggested as an explanation.

In the 1950s, the Chinese government performed thousands of experiments and clinical studies to compare traditional and modern Western medicine, and the traditional system was claimed capable of holding its own.

In a recent trial at Great Ormond Street Hospital for Sick Children, Chinese herbal medicine proved very effective in treating certain types of eczema. Further research studies are currently underway in the UK to investigate its efficacy for asthma, migraine and irritable bowel syndrome.

Rating

Popularity	Medical Credibility	Scientific Research	Availability
✫✫✫	✫✫✫	✫✫✫✫	✫✫✫

VISUALISATION

People who are terrified at the prospect of speaking in public are told to imagine themselves approaching the platform in a calm and confident manner; to see themselves talking eloquently, the audience rapt in admiring concentration, and finally bursting into enthusiastic applause.

Visualisation – the harnessing of the creative power of the imagination – seems to help people deal with difficult situations, and, so a number of doctors and practitioners believe, can activate their own self-healing abilities against physical disease and psychological disorders.

Cancer patients have been encouraged to imagine their healthy disease-fighting white blood cells as white knights on horseback, or as sharp-toothed fish, demolishing a disintegrating rabble of cancer cells. The American cancer specialist, Carl Simonton, and his psychologist wife, Stephanie Matthews-Simonton, who developed these self-help techniques in the 1970s, maintained that patients in their programme lived on average twice as long as others, and, in some cases, that the disease stopped spreading. The extent of these claims has since been disputed, but certainly visualisation seems to help patients feel they have a part to play in tackling their condition, and several distinguished British cancer specialists include it in their treatment.

Absolute relaxation is essential for conjuring up your imaginative skills (see *Relaxation*), and so is choosing the right image. One of Simonton's patients 'saw' his cancer as a powerful black rat and the white cells as rather wimpy eggs sitting in an incubator waiting to hatch. Not surprisingly, perhaps, he was getting worse rather than better. Meanwhile, American surgeon, Dr Bernie Siegel, tries to tap the intuitive power of dream imagery; he encourages his patients to draw pictures that may unconsciously reveal not only their disease, but their attitude towards it.

Doctors say
Psychoneuroimmunology, the newly developing study of the mind – body connection, may offer an explanation of how mental imagery can affect the cells of the immune system. Psychologists also speculate that engaging the creative and intuitive facilities of the right brain hemisphere could balance an unhealthy dominance by the logical, rational left hemisphere, and rally the body's healing forces.

Most conventional practitioners would concede that positive thinking is a useful tool in restoring and maintaining health, but do not expect miracles. Not everybody has a vivid imagination, and an inability to picture cancer-munching sharks is no sign of failure.

Rating

Popularity	Medical Credibility	Scientific Research	Availability
☆☆☆	☆☆☆	☆☆☆	☆☆☆

VOICE THERAPY

How can we sing in the bath with gusto and yet squeak when we address a group of people? The way we speak reveals more about our physical, mental and emotional state than we realise. Lack of confidence, anger, depression, anxiety – these are only some of the conditions reflected in the pace, tone, pitch and rhythm of our voice. Voice movement therapist, Paul Newham, said: 'When we sound good we feel good, and when we feel good we sound good.'

Ambitious women often find themselves sabotaged by a voice that lacks authority; soft, high-pitched and 'feminine', as they were conditioned to speak when young. Years of bad posture, strained breathing from the chest rather than the abdomen, and habitual muscle patterns in the throat and neck can literally throttle our voices, so that we do not sound as we would wish.

Voice therapists – often known as voice movement therapists – use breathing exercises, massage and psychotherapy to help people break through constrictions and inhibitions, and establish a connection between the voice control centre and their emotions. Singing can help the breakthrough: many people, who as children were told not to sing because they were 'out of tune', discover a liberating form of expression.

The voice is a tool of sound (see *Sound therapy*). If high notes shatter glass, what can sound vibrations do to the body? It is no surprise that many traditions, as in India and Tibet, regard sound as a creative force, a bridge between the physical and emotional.

Best for

Those who feel uncomfortable with their voice, lack control of it, or have difficulty expressing their emotions would benefit from such therapy. Those suffering from depression, tension, physical disability and stammering have reported improvement.

What happens

At the initial consultation you will be asked about your health and lifestyle, and then told to make your most effortless natural sound, while the therapist listens to the tones of your voice and observes the muscle tone of your body. Because the aim is to release feelings and emotions which may have become blocked, the therapist will not worry about pronunciation or tune, but will try to improve the *sounds* you make, and, as you continue to vocalise, will massage and manipulate your body, suggesting ways of moving, moods to express, and images to conjure up that will affect your voice. Sessions last an hour and cost from £15 to £40, depending on the therapist's experience.

Doctors say

Voice movement therapy is not widely available or well known, but there is no reason why it should not benefit stress-related conditions, especially if breathing problems or emotional distress are factors.

Rating

Popularity	Medical Credibility	Scientific Research	Availability
✷	✷✷	✷	✷✷

YOGA

The weekly yoga class in the school or church hall has become part of the British way of life. There are more than 5000 teachers and over half a million people in the UK practising yoga regularly, though it is probably fair to say that most see it as a way of keeping fit and supple, without giving a great deal of thought to the philosophy behind it.

Going by ancient carvings, yoga – the word is from the Sanskrit for 'union,' and has the same root as the English 'yoke' – was practised in India as long as 6000 years ago. Spiritual, mental and physical exercises were designed to lead the practitioner into a mystical harmony with higher consciousness.

There are several forms of yoga; some, such as Raja and Jnana, focus on spiritual and mental integration. Hatha yoga, the form most common in modern Britain and the most comfortable for Western minds, is mainly concerned with physical postures, known as *asanas*, and breathing, or *pranayama*. It became popular during the 1960s, partly through the general interest in Eastern mysticism fuelled by the Beatles and the Maharishi Mahesh Yogi, and partly through the efforts of followers such as the violinist Yehudi Menuhin, who claimed that yoga helped cure his 'frozen' shoulder. His teacher, B.K.S. Iyengar, had developed a particularly strong form of hatha yoga that is widely taught today.

Almost anybody, young and old, can benefit from yoga exercises. Movements and postures are co-ordinated with inhalation and exhalation of the breath (seen as the embodiment of *prana*, or the life force), and performed slowly and deliberately, mind and body focused in a concentrated awareness that is a kind of meditation. Many of the poses, such as the Dog, the Cobra and the Ostrich, are borrowed from the unselfconsciously relaxed attitudes of animals.

Best for

Keeping fit and supple for those in good health; increasingly recognised as therapeutic for those with stress-related conditions, fatigue, headaches and migraine, depression, ME (myalgic encephalomyelitis), high blood pressure and heart disorders, rheumatoid arthritis, digestive disorders, premenstrual syndrome, asthma, back problems and pain relief (anyone suffering from these conditions should inform the teacher so that appropriate exercises can be done). Special classes for handicapped people report benefits, such as increased flexibility, relaxation and improved concentration.

What happens

Daily practice at home will increase any benefits, but ideally, to begin with, you should find a teacher rather than trying to learn from books. Classes usually last 60 to 90 minutes, and fees vary according to where you live and how many are in the class. Wear loose, comfortable clothing and go barefoot. A rug or rubber mat is advisable to stop you slipping on the floor. There is no sense of competition, and you will be encouraged to go at your own pace. Most classes end with five or ten minutes relaxation in the 'corpse' pose, flat on your back on the floor.

Doctors say

Yoga is not a controversial pursuit, though many would regard it as a leisure activity and be less aware of its therapeutic benefits. Check with your GP if you plan to take up yoga and are taking any medication or suffer from a heart condition, back pain or joint problems. Yoga combines stretching exercises, now seen as an essential part of fitness in sports medicine, and breathing, relaxation and meditation techniques. A mass of research evidence shows the latter can lower blood pressure and slow the metabolic rate. In a recent study at Oxford University, yoga proved more effective in restoring energy than either relaxation or visualisation.

Rating

Popularity	Medical Credibility	Scientific Research	Availability
✫✫✫✫	✫✫✫	✫✫✫✫	✫✫✫✫

COMMON AILMENTS

The following is a list of common ailments and the complementary treatments that might be appropriate, once you have consulted your GP. Many of them are self-help treatments; health stores and some pharmacists have information about over-the-counter homeopathic and herbal remedies. A number of books are available which list self-help techniques for various treatments (see *Further reading* on page 175). For information on how to find a qualified practitioner see page 143.

ACNE   herbalism, homeopathy, nutritional therapy

ALLERGIC DERMATITIS   (a rash on the skin in reaction to a substance) clinical ecology, kinesiology

ALLERGIES: (FOOD)   clinical ecology, kinesiology naturopathy, nutritional therapy

ALLERGIES: (HAY FEVER)   acupressure, aromatherapy, clinical ecology, homeopathy, kinesiology, nutritional therapy

ANAEMIA   acupuncture, biochemic tissue salts, nutritional therapy, traditional Chinese medicine

ANKYLOSING SPONDYLITIS   (inflammatory disease of the spine and pelvis): acupuncture, aromatherapy, chiropractic, homeopathy, hydrotherapy, massage, osteopathy, yoga

ANXIETY   aromatherapy, Bach flower remedies, biofeedback, herbalism, massage, meditation, nutritional therapy, psychotherapy and counselling, relaxation, traditional Chinese medicine, yoga

ARTHRITIS (OSTEOARTHRITIS)   acupuncture, Alexander technique, hydrotherapy, massage, naturopathy, nutritional therapy, osteopathy, traditional Chinese medicine

ASTHMA   acupressure, aromatherapy, clinical ecology, herbalism, homeopathy, nutritional therapy, osteopathy, reflexology, traditional Chinese medicine, yoga

BACKACHE   acupressure, acupuncture, Alexander Technique, chiropractic, hydrotherapy, massage, osteopathy, relaxation

BOILS   aromatherapy, biochemic tissue salts, herbalism, homeopathy, traditional Chinese medicine

BRONCHITIS   aromatherapy, herbalism, homeopathy, traditional Chinese medicine

BRUISES   Bach flower remedies, herbalism, homeopathy, hydrotherapy

CANCER   (no complementary medicine or therapy can claim to cure cancer, but they may offer an alleviation of pain and a more positive outlook) homeopathy, massage, naturopathy, psychotherapy and counselling, reflexology, relaxation, visualisation

COLDS   aromatherapy, herbalism, homeopathy, nutritional therapy

COLD SORES   aromatherapy, homeopathy, nutritional therapy

COLITIS   acupressure, clinical ecology, herbalism, homeopathy

CONSTIPATION   acupressure, Bach flower remedies, colonic irrigation, massage, naturopathy, nutritional therapy, yoga

CYSTITIS   aromatherapy, herbalism, homeopathy, hydrotherapy, nutritional therapy

DEPRESSION   aromatherapy, Bach flower remedies, psychotherapy and counselling

ECZEMA   acupressure, clinical ecology, herbalism, homeopathy, relaxation, traditional Chinese medicine

FATIGUE   acupuncture, aromatherapy, Bach flower remedies, homeopathy, naturopathy, relaxation, yoga

FEET, ACHING   aromatherapy, chiropractic, massage, osteopathy, reflexology

FIBROSITIS   acupressure, acupuncture, Alexander Technique, aromatherapy, chiropractic, homeopathy, hydrotherapy, massage, meditation, osteopathy, relaxation, yoga

FLUID RETENTION   acupressure, aromatherapy, herbalism, massage, tissue salts

FROZEN SHOULDER   acupressure, acupuncture, Alexander Technique, chiropractic, hydrotherapy, osteopathy, massage

GASTRITIS herbalism, homeopathy, nutritional therapy, relaxation

HAEMORRHOIDS herbalism, homeopathy, hydrotherapy, massage, naturopathy, nutritional therapy

HEADACHE acupressure, acupuncture, Alexander Technique, aromatherapy, chiropractic, herbalism, homeopathy, massage, osteopathy

HEARTBURN herbalism, homeopathy, nutritional therapy, traditional Chinese medicine

HIGH BLOOD PRESSURE acupressure, aromatherapy, herbalism, homeopathy, massage, relaxation, traditional Chinese medicine, yoga

HIVES clinical ecology, herbalism, homeopathy, kinesiology

IMPOTENCE acupressure, aromatherapy, massage, meditation, psychotherapy and counselling, relaxation, traditional Chinese medicine, yoga

INFERTILITY homeopathy, relaxation, traditional Chinese medicine

INFLAMMATORY BOWEL DISEASE clinical ecology, herbalism, homeopathy, naturopathy, nutritional therapy

INSECT BITES AND STINGS aromatherapy, Bach flower remedies, biochemic tissue salts, herbalism, homeopathy

INSOMNIA acupressure, aromatherapy, herbalism, homeopathy, relaxation, traditional Chinese medicine

IRRITABLE BOWEL SYNDROME aromatherapy, biofeedback, herbalism, homeopathy, nutritional therapy, relaxation, traditional Chinese medicine, yoga

ME (MYALGIC ENCEPHALOMYELITIS) (also known as post-viral fatigue syndrome and chronic fatigue syndrome) acupuncture, autogenic training, biofeedback, clinical ecology, herbalism, homeopathy, meditation, naturopathy, nutritional therapy, relaxation, yoga

MENOPAUSAL PROBLEMS acupuncture, herbalism, homeopathy, naturopathy, nutritional therapy, psychotherapy and counselling

MIGRAINE   acupressure, acupuncture, aromatherapy, clinical ecology, chiropractic, herbalism, homeopathy, kinesiology, osteopathy, reflexology, relaxation, yoga

NECK PAIN AND STIFFNESS   acupressure, Alexander Technique, chiropractic, massage, osteopathy, reflexology, relaxation, yoga

NEURALGIA   acupuncture, aromatherapy, chiropractic, herbalism, homeopathy, hypnotherapy, osteopathy, traditional Chinese medicine

ORAL THRUSH (*Candida albicans*)   herbalism, homeopathy, naturopathy, nutritional therapy

OSTEOPOROSIS AND ASSOCIATED DISCOMFORT   acupuncture, herbalism, naturopathy, osteopathy, traditional Chinese medicine

PAIN   acupressure, acupuncture, aromatherapy, hypnotherapy, massage, relaxation, spiritual healing, visualisation

PANIC ATTACK   aromatherapy, Bach flower remedies, herbalism, homeopathy, hypnotherapy, meditation, psychotherapy and counselling, relaxation, yoga

PELVIC INFLAMMATORY DISEASE (orthodox treatment with antibiotics is essential)   herbalism, homeopathy, hydrotherapy

PEPTIC ULCER   biofeedback, herbalism, homeopathy, massage, meditation, naturopathy, relaxation, traditional Chinese medicine, yoga

PERIOD PAIN   acupressure, acupuncture, aromatherapy, biochemic tissue salts, herbalism, homeopathy, massage, osteopathy, traditional Chinese medicine, yoga

PERIODS, HEAVY   herbalism, homeopathy, naturopathy

PHOBIA   aromatherapy, Bach flower remedies, biofeedback, herbalism, hypnotherapy, meditation, naturopathy, behavioural psychotherapy, relaxation, visualisation, yoga

POSTNATAL DEPRESSION   acupuncture, herbalism, homeopathy, naturopathy, osteopathy

PREMENSTRUAL SYNDROME (PMS)   acupuncture, homeopathy, meditation, osteopathy, relaxation, traditional Chinese medicine, yoga

PSORIASIS   clinical ecology, herbalism, homeopathy, hydrotherapy, kinesiology, naturopathy, traditional Chinese medicine

RHEUMATOID ARTHRITIS   acupuncture, chiropractic, herbalism, homeopathy, hydrotherapy, massage, naturopathy, nutritional therapy, osteopathy, traditional Chinese medicine

SCIATICA   acupressure, acupuncture, chiropractic, massage, osteopathy

SEASONAL AFFECTIVE DISORDER (SAD)   light therapy, naturopathy, relaxation

SEX DRIVE PROBLEMS   acupressure, aromatherapy, psychotherapy and counselling

SINUSITIS   acupressure, clinical ecology, herbalism, homeopathy, hydrotherapy, naturopathy, osteopathy, traditional Chinese medicine

SPRAINS   acupuncture, aromatherapy, chiropractic, homeopathy, hydrotherapy, massage, osteopathy

STRESS   acupuncture, aromatherapy, autogenic training, biofeedback, shiatsu, traditional Chinese medicine, massage, meditation, psychotherapy and counselling, relaxation, yoga

THRUSH   (*Candida albicans*): aromatherapy, naturopathy, nutritional therapy

TINNITIS   acupressure, acupuncture, cranial osteopathy, homeopathy, naturopathy, yoga

TRAVEL SICKNESS   acupressure, aromatherapy, Bach flower remedies, herbalism, homeopathy

VAGINAL IRRITATION   aromatherapy, herbalism, naturopathy

WARTS   herbalism, homeopathy, hypnotherapy, visualisation

WHIPLASH INJURY   acupressure, acupuncture, aromatherapy, Alexander Technique, chiropractic, homeopathy, massage, osteopathy

FINDING A QUALIFIED PRACTITIONER

Contact these professional organisations and registering bodies to find a qualified practitioner in each of the different therapies and treatments. If you are outside the UK, look in the phone book under the name of the treatment or therapy.

ACUPRESSURE

The Shen Tao Foundation, Middle Piccadilly Natural Healing Centre, Holwell, Sherborne, Dorset DT9 5LW. Tel. (0963) 23468. Shiatsu practitioners include acupressure in their treatment. Contact The Shiatsu Society, 5 Foxcote, Wokingham, Berks RG11 3PG. Tel. (0734) 730 836.

ACUPUNCTURE

It is important to consult an acupuncturist who is a member of one of the five bodies associated with the Council for Acupuncture. This forum maintains high standards of ethics, discipline and codes of practice, education and training through the British Acupuncture Accreditation Board (BAAB) – an independent body regulating qualifications; courses must be a minimum of two years full-time, and include Western medical training in anatomy, physiology and pathology. It also promotes further research, and publishes a Directory of British Acupuncturists, which combines the registers of member associations. Copies are available from the Council for Acupuncture, 179 Gloucester Place, London NW1 6DX. Tel (071) 724 5756.

Member associations are: The British Acupuncture Association and Register (the initials MBAAR and FBAAR stand for Member and Fellow of the BAAR); the International Register of Oriental Medicine UK (MIROM); the Register of Traditional Chinese Medicine (MRTCM); the Traditional Acupuncture Society (MTAS); and the Chung San Acupuncture Society (CSAS). If thumbing through the Yellow Pages for a local practitioner, look for the qualifications LicAc (Licentiate in Acupuncture), DipAc (Diploma of Acupuncture) or BAc (Bachelor of Acupuncture) before the letters of the professional associations.

For a list of medical doctors who have trained in acupuncture, contact the British Medical Acupuncture Society, Newton House Newton Lane, Lower Whitley, Warrington, Cheshire WA4 4JA. Tel (0925) 730 727.

ALEXANDER TECHNIQUE

All teachers of the Alexander Technique should complete a three-year course at a training school recognised by the Society of Teachers of the Alexander Technique (STAT). This entitles them to use the initials STAT, but many do not seem to bother. For the name of a teacher in your area, write (with sae) to the Society of Teachers of the Alexander Technique, 20 London House, 266 Fulham Road, London SW10 9EL. Tel (071) 351 0828.

ANTHROPOSOPHICAL MEDICINE

Anthroposophical Medical Association, c/o Rudolf Steiner House 35 Park Road, London NW1 6XT. Tel (071) 723 4400.

Many of the specialised treatments are available at an anthroposophical therapeutic centre in the Park Attwood Clinic Trimpley, Bewdley, Worcestershire DY12 1RE. Tel (0299) 861444.

AROMATHERAPY

It is important to consult a fully trained aromatherapist. The Aromatherapy Organisations Council (AOC) has set a minimum training standard of 180 hours in a class which includes lessons in massage, anatomy and physiology. For a list of member associations, contact the Aromatherapy Organisations Council, 3 Latymer Close, Braybrooke, Market Harborough, Leicester LE16 8LN. Tel (0858) 434242.

ART THERAPY

A two-year, full-time postgraduate diploma course in art therapy is available at several colleges. Full members of the British Association of Art Therapists (BAAT) are known as Registered Art Therapists (RATh). For information, contact the British Association of Art Therapists, 11a Brighton Road, Brighton BN2 3RL.

AURA HEALING

Not all healers work with the aura, but some do, and for further information, contact the National Federation of Spiritual Healers Old Manor Farm Studio, Church Street, Sunbury-on-Thames, Middlesex TW16 6RG. Tel (0932) 783 164.

AUTOGENIC TRAINING

Practitioners are usually doctors, psychologists, psychotherapists and nurses who complete a two-year, part-time training. For further information and a list of practitioners, write (with sae) to Mrs Jane Bird, Hon. Sec., British Association for Autogenic Training and Therapy (BAFATT), 18 Holtsmere Close Garston, Watford, Herts WD2 6NG. Tel (0923) 675 501.

AYURVEDIC MEDICINE

Until about fifteen years ago in India, ayurvedic medicine was poorly regulated, and there were quacks and badly trained practitioners in abundance, although it remained the healthcare most accessible for the majority of Indians. Now, a Central Council for Ayurveda keeps an eye on training and practice; colleges attached to universities offer a five and a half-year degree course (Bachelor of Ayurvedic Surgery and Medicine) which includes a basic study of Western medicine. For further information, write (with sae) to the International Association of Ayurveda, PO Box 3043, Barnet, Herts EN4 0QZ.

Fees are about £70 for an initial session, then £35 for four- to six-monthly seasonal consultations.

BACH FLOWER REMEDIES

For further information, contact The Bach Centre, Mount Vernon, Sotwell, Wallingford, Oxon OX10 0PZ. Tel (0491) 834678.

THE BATES METHOD

Teachers should all be members of the Bates Association of Great Britain. For a list of teachers, write (with sae) to: Bates Association of Great Britain, Friars Court, 11 Tarmount Lane, Shoreham by Sea, West Sussex BN43 6RQ.

BIOCHEMIC TISSUE SALTS

See *Homeopathy*, *Naturopathy* and *Herbalism*.

BIOENERGETICS

There are very few practitioners: Guy Gladstone runs individual and group sessions, contact: Open Centre, 188 Old Street, London EC1V 9FR. Tel (081) 549 9583.

Fees range from £25, for an initial hour-long session, to £30 for a day's group session, and £60 for a weekend group. For training enquiries, contact Maggie Taraz, the British Association of Analytical Body Psychotherapy, Tel (0273) 303 382.

For biodynamics, a form of bioenergetics, contact the Gerda Boyesen Centre, Acacia House, Centre Avenue, Acton Park, London W3 7JX. Tel (081) 746 0499. Fees are £25 to £30 for an hour's session. Training is a three-year course, followed by two years of supervised practice before registration.

BIOFEEDBACK

Finding a trained supervisor and equipment is difficult, as most machines and the people who know how to use them are attached to hospitals and universities. Also, people have found it hard to reproduce at home the sensations that they mastered in the laboratory.

Portable machines for home use are available, at prices ranging from £70 (Ultramind's *RelaxPlus* software for IBM-compatible computers with a mouse is about £200) but you cannot just plug in and say 'I will relax', because often the opposite happens. Learning some *relaxation, visualisation* or *meditation* techniques beforehand will help to get started.

Workshops on these techniques, and the use of home equipment, are run by the Maxwell Cade Foundation, 9 Chatsworth Road, London NW2 4BJ. Tel (081) 749 3983/451 0083. (Cade, a biophysicist, pioneered biofeedback in the UK.)

BIORHYTHMS

In theory, it is not difficult to work out your biorhythm cycles, provided you know your date of birth and have a computer or calculator programmed to do the job. Alternatively, various companies that advertise in newspapers and magazines will undertake it for you – at a price.

CHIROPRACTIC

A five-year B.Sc. Honours course, and one-year postgraduate training at the Anglo-European College of Chiropractic in Bournemouth make chiropractic the longest and highest qualified alternative therapy course in the UK. Graduates will use B.Sc. Chiropractic after their name, but older practitioners, who qualified before the introduction of the degree course in 1991, have DC (Diploma in Chiropractic). Australian chiropractors use the letters BAppSci (Bachelor of Applied Science) Chiropractic.

A Parliamentary Act is expected to regulate chiropractic later this year, but in the meantime anybody can still call themselves 'chiropractors'. Manipulating the spine can go disastrously wrong, so it is vital to check that the practitioner is properly qualified. Members of the British Chiropractic Association (MBCA) must abide by the rules and code of ethics and practice of the Association.

For a list of qualified chiropractors, contact the British Chiropractic Association, 29 Whitley Street, Reading, Berks RG2 0EG. Tel (0734) 757 557. Scottish Chiropractic Association, 46 Richmond Street, Aberdeen, AB2 4TR. Tel (0224) 635550. Or telephone Freephone 0800 212 618 to make an appointment with the chiropractor nearest to you.

McTimoney Chiropractic

Institute of Pure Chiropractic (McTimoney), 14 Park End Street, Oxford OX1 1HH. Tel (0865) 246 687. Graduates of the Witney School of Chiropractics (McTimoney-Corley practitioners) belong to British Association of Applied Chiropractic, 3 Meadows Close, Skipton under Wychwood, Oxford OX7 6BY. Tel (0869) 321 166.

CLINICAL ECOLOGY

Clinical ecologists should always be medically trained so that serious diseases are not overlooked. You will need a referral from your GP, so ask your doctor to contact the British Society for Allergy and Environmental Medicine with the British Society for Nutritional Medicine, Acorns, Romsey Road, Cadnam, Southampton SO4 2NN. Further information can be obtained from Action Against Allergy, 24–26 High Street, Hampton Hill, Middlesex TW12 1PD.

COLONIC IRRIGATION

Colonic irrigation can be dangerous in untrained hands, so contact the Colonic International Association, 50A Morrish Road, London SW2 4EG.

COLOUR THERAPY

Most practitioners take part-time courses through one of the following organisations. For names of practitioners contact Living Colour, 33 Lancaster Grove, London NW3 4EX. Tel (071) 794 1371). International Association for Colour Therapy (IACT), PO Box 3688, London SW13 0NX. Tel (081) 878 5276. Hygeia College of Colour Therapy, Theo Gimbel, Brook House, Avening, Tetbury, Glos. GL8 8NS. Tel (0453) 832 150.

CRANIAL OSTEOPATHY

All osteopaths will have to be registered with the General Osteopathic Council (GOsC) after 1997, a statutory body which will oversee the profession's standard of training, clinical skill and professional conduct.

For qualified practitioners specialising in cranial osteopathy contact the Osteopathic Information Service, PO Box 2074, Reading, Berkshire RG1 4YR. Please enclose an sae. Sutherland Cranial College (0432) 356655; or, if the patient is a child, the Osteopathic Centre for Children (071) 495 1231.

CRANIO-SACRAL THERAPY

Cranio-sacral practitioners are not trained osteopaths (and indeed are not necessarily qualified in anything), although many are practising aromatherapists and massage practitioners. Courses are run by the College of Cranio-Sacral Therapy (Tel. 0622 729231) and the Craniosacral Therapy Educational Trust (Tel. 081 349 0297).

CRYSTAL AND GEM HEALING

A number of crystal healing organisations, under the umbrella of the Affiliation of Crystal Healing Organisations (ACHO), a member of the BCMA (British Complementary Medicine Association), have agreed a minimum training period and group insurance scheme. For information, send a stamped addressed envelope to the Affiliation of

149

Crystal Healing Organisations, 46 Lower Green, Esher KT10 8HD.
Tel (081) 398 7252.

DANCE MOVEMENT THERAPY

Anyone suffering from a physical, mental or emotional disorder
should find a qualified dance therapist, who is trained in handling
these conditions. Contact the Association for Dance Movement
Therapy, c/o The Arts Therapies Department, Springfield Hospital,
Glenburnie Road, London SW17 7DJ. Otherwise, it is a case of trial
and error. Dance movement classes are sometimes advertised in
local libraries and magazines.

DO-IN

A few initial lessons are a good idea to ensure you are going in the
right direction. Contact the Community Health Foundation, 188
Old Street, London EC1V 9BP.

THE FELDENKRAIS METHOD

There is a four-year, part-time training for practitioners; for a list,
contact the Feldenkrais Guild UK, PO Box 370, London N10 3XA.
Regular classes are held at the Open Centre, 188 Old Street,
London EC1V 9BP.

FLOATATION THERAPY

There are a growing number of tanks throughout the UK. The
average charge is £10-£20 per session. Send a stamped addressed
envelope and £1 in envelope marked 'Centres' to the Floatation
Tank Association, PO Box 168, Rickmansworth, Herts WD3 5TY.
Tel (0923) 285 868. The training course for FTA members is a one
day course.

FLOWER AND GEM ESSENCES

Clare Harvey, of the International Federation of Vibrational
Medicine, practises at Middle Piccadilly Natural Healing Centre,
Holwell, Sherborne, Dorset DT9 5LW. Tel (0963) 23468 and The
Hale Clinic, 7 Park Crescent, London W1N 3HE. Tel (071) 631
0156. For other practitioners, contact the Flower and Gem Remedy
Association, Laurel Farm Clinic, 17 Carlingcott Peasetown St John
Bath BA2 8AN. Tel (0761) 434 098.

HEALING

It is thought that about three-quarters of us have healing gifts. Some
may find them easier to develop than others, although most people
would probably be too embarrassed to try. Not uncommonly, people
say they found they could heal after experiencing some great
trauma, a critical illness or bereavement.

Commander David Repard, chairman of the Confederation of
Healing Organisations (CHO), which represents several thousand
healers registered in 12 member groups, is working on a system
of NVQs (National Vocational Qualifications). Meanwhile, those
wishing to become acknowledged healers can enrol with one of
the member organisations, all of which are registered charities.
Entry is strictly controlled, and training involves two years as a
probationer under the supervision of an experienced healer.
Qualification involves, among other things, references from
four patients who believe they have benefited.

The CHO has always seen itself as truly 'complementary,' working
alongside conventional practitioners. Members of the CHO adhere
to a code of conduct drawn up after informal consultation with
members of the General Medical Council, the British Medical
Association and the Royal Colleges of Medicine, significant
elements of which were later incorporated in the British
Complementary Medicine Association's code of practice.
Registered healers are covered by insurance only as long
as they keep within this code.

The code of conduct forbids medical diagnoses by healers unless they are doctors, or the treatment of a child without a parent's permission. If they suspect a serious condition, they must advise you to see your GP. Registered healers will not promise cures, go into trance, ask you to take your clothes off, practise clairvoyance, take you into past lives, hypnotise you or do anything extreme. Women seeing a male healer can request that a third person be present.

Many healers do not charge a fee. Most appreciate a donation but leave it up to you to decide how much to give. Some refuse to take anything at all because they feel it would be a misuse of their gift from God. Where there are outgoing expenses, such as rents and overheads, the healer may be obliged to charge in order to survive. Ask beforehand whether there is a fee and, if so, how much. It is usually £15 to £20, perhaps more in an expensive area. Avoid healers who charge excessively or promise miracles; greed and healing do not go hand in hand.

For general information contact the Confederation of Healing Organisations, Suite J, 2nd Floor, The Red and White House, 113 High Street, Berkhamsted, Herts HP4 2DJ. Tel (0442) 870 660.

To find a CHO healer, contact the following member organisations: Spiritualist Association of Great Britain, 33 Belgrave Square, London W1. Tel (071) 235 3351.

For spiritual healing: The British Alliance of Healing Associations, 26 Highfield Avenue, Herne Bay, Kent CT6 6LM. Tel (0227) 373 804.

Non-denominational: The College of Healing, 3 Runnings Park, Croft Bank, West Malvern, Worcs. Tel (0684) 565 253. Maitreya School of Healing, 2 Jeymer Avenue, London NW2 4PL. Tel (081) 452 2882. The National Federation of Spiritual Healers, Old Manor Farm Studio, Church Street, Sunbury on Thames, Middlesex TW16 6RG. Tel (0932) 783164/5. World Federation of Healing, 9 Gallards Close, London Road, Southborough, Tunbridge Wells, Kent TN4 0NB. Tel (0892) 514 342. Association of Therapeutic Healers, Flat 5, Neal Street, Covent Garden, London WC2. Tel (071) 240 0176. The College of Psychic Studies, The College, 16 Queensberry Place, London SW7 2EB. Tel (071) 589 3292. The Fellowship of Erasmus, Moat House, Banyard's Green, Laxfield, Woodbridge,

Suffolk IP13 8ER. Tel (0986) 798 682. Sufi Healing Order of Great Britain, 29 Grosvenor Place, London Road, Bath, Avon BA6 6BA. Tel (0225) 312 694.

Non-denominational distant healing: The Radionics Association, Baerlein House, Goose Green, Deddington, Banbury, Oxon OX15 0SZ. Tel (0869) 38852.

Non-denominational Christian: The White Eagle Lodge, Brewells Lane, Rake, Liss, Hants GU33 7HY. Tel (0730) 893 300.

HERBALISM

A four year B.Sc. degree course for medical herbalists is now in its final stages of validation at a British university. Current practitioners have completed a four-year course at the School of Herbal Medicine (Phytotherapy) in East Sussex, and are members of the National Institute of Medical Herbalists (NIMH), using the letters MNIMH or FNIMH. A member of the Council for Complementary and Alternative Medicine (CCAM), the Institute has a code of ethics, a disciplinary framework and a register of practitioners. For a list of local herbalists, send a stamped addressed envelope to the National Institute of Medical Herbalists, 9 Palace Gate, Exeter, Devon EX1 1JA.

The General Council and Register of Consultant Herbalists offers a correspondence course. Graduates use the letters MRH or FRH. The Council's address is Grosvenor House, 40 Sea Way, Middleton-on-Sea, West Sussex PO22 7SA.

HOMEOPATHY

More than 600 doctors have taken a postgraduate training course to become a Member or Fellow of the Faculty of Homeopathy (MFHom and FFHom). Many are in private practice, although a few work in the National Health Service. There are five NHS homeopathic hospitals – in London, Glasgow, Bristol, Liverpool and Tunbridge Wells. For further information and a list of registered homeopaths send a large stamped addressed envelope to the British

Homeopathic Association, 27a Devonshire Street, London W1N 1RJ. Tel (071) 935 2163.

Non-medically qualified homeopaths can register with the Society of Homeopaths after completing a four-year training course at an accredited college, followed by at least one year's clinical supervision. The society has a code of ethics. Send a large stamped addressed envelope for a list of registered homeopaths to the Society of Homeopaths, 2 Artizan Road, Northampton NN1 4HU. Tel (0604) 21400. Further information is also available from the Hahnemann Society, 2 Powis Place, Great Ormond Street, London WC1N 3HT. Tel (071) 837 3297.

HYDROTHERAPY

It is expensive, but a few days at a health farm can introduce you to hydrotherapy of one sort or another.

Many naturopaths are skilled in hydrotherapy. Contact the British Naturopathic and Osteopathic Association, Frazer House, 6 Netherhall Gardens, London NW3 5RR.

Your GP may refer you to an NHS or recommended private physiotherapist, if it is felt that your condition would benefit from this therapy.

HYPNOTHERAPY

Anyone can advertise themselves as a hypnotherapist, or offer correspondence courses with 'diplomas' and a string of letters that are pure fantasy. Protect yourself by checking any health problems with your GP, who may be able to refer you to an NHS psychologist practising hypnosis. Seek a practitioner through a professional body, not the telephone directory or local paper. Beware of someone who promises cures or tries to make you pay for several sessions in advance. Fees should average £25-£35 for an hour.

For details of members of the Association of Hypnotherapy Organisations (AHO) contact the British Complementary Medicine Association Tel.(081) 964 1205) or the AHO chairman Nick Garrett, 6a Portsmouth Road, Woolston, Southampton, Hants SO2

9AA. Tel (0703) 438 157. Two organisations which are BCMA members and have their own code of practice and register of practitioners, are: British Hypnosis Research, The Burleigh Business Centre, 52 Burleigh Street, Cambridge CB1 1DJ. Tel (0223) 350 012. Practitioners tend to be members of the caring professions who take a 30-day diploma course over five years.

The National Society for Hypnotherapists and Psychotherapists (NSHAP) (Tel. (071) 226 6963) publishes the Central Register of Advanced Hypnotherapists (CRAH) (one year, part-time, NSHAP diploma course followed by two years clinical supervision). Write to the Registrar, CRAH, 28 Finsbury Park Road, London N4 2JX.

For doctors and dentists using hypnosis, contact the British Society of Medical and Dental Hypnosis (BSMDH), National Office 17 Keppelview Road, Kimberworth, Rotherham SG1 2AR. Tel (0709) 554 558. BSMDH Metropolitan and South, 42 Links Road, Ashtead, Surrey KT21 2HJ. Tel (0372) 273 522. BSMDH Scotland, PO Box 1007, Glasgow G31 2LE, Tel./fax (041) 556 1606.

For psychologists and doctors using hypnosis, contact the British Society of Experimental and Clinical Hypnosis, c/o Dr Michael Heap, University of Sheffield Centre for Psychotherapeutic Studies, 16 Claremont Crescent, Sheffield S10 2TA. Tel (0742) 824 970.

IRIDOLOGY

Practitioners who have completed a 12 to 18-month training course are registered with the National Council and Register of Iridologists, 998 Winborne Road, Bournemouth BH9 2DE. Tel (0202) 518 078 and use the letters MBRI (Member of the British Register of Iridologists). Send stamped addressed envelope for further information.

KINESIOLOGY

Practitioners complete at least 150 hours training and 200 hours clinical experience within two years. For further information and a list of practitioners, send stamped addressed envelope to the Kinesiology Federation/Touch For Health, 30 Sudley Road,

Bognor Regis, West Sussex PO21 1ER. Tel (0243) 841 689 or
the Association for Systematic Kinesiology, 39 Browns Road,
Surbiton, KT5 8ST. Tel (081) 399 3215.

Systematic Kinesiology includes all variations of kinesiology, such
as behavioural, clinical and educational kinesiology. Classes in
Touch For Health, a gentle form of self-help kinesiology for lay
people, are available through the Association. A number of
practitioners qualified in other fields, such as osteopaths,
chiropractors, physiotherapists, naturopaths, homeopaths and
herbalists, practise kinesiology.

LIGHT THERAPY

For further information and a list of light box suppliers send a large
stamped addressed envelope to the SAD Association, Box 989,
London SW7 2PZ.

MASSAGE

Some people call themselves massage practitioners after two or
three weekends of training, and there are many training colleges and
organisations. The newly-formed British Massage Therapy Council
is an umbrella group that aims to organise, and develop minimum
training standards. As a member of the British Complementary
Medicine Association (BCMA), it has a code of ethics and
complaints procedure. For further information contact the British
Massage Therapy Council, 3 Woodhouse Cliff, Headingley, Leeds
L56 2HF. Tel (0532) 785 601.

ITEC (International Therapy Examinations Council) is a nationally
recognised qualification in anatomy, physiology and massage. For
names of practitioners with this diploma contact the Institute for
Complementary Medicine, PO Box 194, London SE16 1QZ. Tel
(071) 237 5165.

For further information about massage send a stamped addressed
envelope to the Clare Maxwell-Hudson School of Massage, PO Box
457, London NW2 4BR.

MEDITATION

There are a number of meditation schools, such as those teaching Transcendental Meditation, but they often involve the adoption of a particular philosophy and even behaviour, which is fine if you are comfortable with it. Although people have managed to start meditating on their own, it can be difficult to discipline yourself at first. Find a group if you can; those practising the basic techniques are becoming more popular, and sometimes they are advertised in local libraries.

METAMORPHIC TECHNIQUE

Practitioners need no qualifications other than attending courses run by the Metamorphic Association. For further information, and the names of practitioners in your area, contact The Metamorphic Association, 67 Ritherdon Road, London SW17 8QE.
Tel (081) 672 5951.

MUSIC THERAPY

There are only a few hundred music therapists in the UK, most working within the NHS and education service, although a few are in private practice. Fees range from £20 to £25 but are negotiable. Therapists must be trained musicians with a degree or diploma from a recognised college, followed by a year's postgraduate course, and they use the letters RMTh (Registered Music Therapist) or SRMTh (State Registered Music Therapist).

For names of therapists, send a stamped addressed envelope to the Coordinator, The Association of Professional Music Therapists, 38 Pierce Lane, Fulbourn, Cambs CB1 5DL or The Administrator, The British Society for Music Therapy, 25 Rosslyn Avenue, East Barnet, Herts EN4 8DH. Tel (081) 368 8879.

NATUROPATHY

As with many therapies and disciplines, anyone can call themselves a naturopath. Look for practitioners who have completed a four-year, full-time course at the British College of Naturopathy and Osteopathy. Graduates hold a Naturopathic Diploma (ND) and as members of the Register of Naturopaths use the letters MRN. For a list of qualified practitioners, write to the General Council and Register of Naturopaths, at the British Naturopathic and Osteopathic Association, Frazer House, 6 Netherhall Gardens, London NW3 5RR.

NUTRITIONAL THERAPY

At the moment, anyone can call themselves a 'nutritional therapist'. Several independent colleges offer part-time training over two years that includes some biochemistry, physiology and nutrition, and one three-month, full-time course is available.

The Society for the Promotion of Nutritional Therapy maintains a directory of practitioners, who have either qualified in other therapies, such as osteopathy, or are graduates of colleges approved by the Society. It is currently establishing a code of practice and will investigate any complaints. For a list of practitioners, send a stamped addressed envelope and £1 to the Society for the Promotion of Nutritional Therapy, First Floor, The Enterprise Centre, Station Parade, Eastbourne BN21 1BE. Tel (0323) 430 203.

Hospital dietitians can advise on an apporpriate diet for your condition. A number of doctors specialising in nutritional medicine practise privately; ask your GP to contact the British Society for Allergy and Environmental Medicine with the British of Nutritional Medicine, Acorns, Romsey Road, Cadnam, Southampton, Hants SO4 2NN.

OSTEOPATHY

When the 1993 Osteopathy Act comes into force (probably in 1997), nobody will be able to call themelves an osteopath unless registered with the new regulatory body, the General Osteopathic Council (GOsC). All osteopaths will have to meet certain standards of training, subscribe to the Council's code of ethics for practitioners, and carry insurance. Until then, as it is still legally possible for an untrained person to practise as an osteopath, it is vital to consult a practitioner who is a member of one of the following four organisations maintaining registers of members. General Council and Register of Osteopaths, 56 London Street, Reading, Berkshire RG1 4SQ. Tel (0734) 576 585/566 260.

Of British practitioners, 75 per cent belong to this organisation. Look for the letters MRO and the title Registered Osteopath. For the name of your nearest Registered Osteopath, contact the Secretary at the above address.

The College of Osteopaths Practitioners Association, 13 Furzhill Road, Borehamwood, Herts WD6 2DG. Tel. (081) 905 1237. Guild of Osteopaths, 181 Erith Road, Bexleyheath, Kent DA7 6HS. Tel (0322) 551 024. British and European Osteopathic Association, c/o Station Road, Sidcup, Kent DA15 7EN. Tel (081) 977 8532.

Osteopathic Information Service, PO Box 2074, Reading, Berkshire RG1 4YR (enclose SAE). Tel. (0734) 512051.

The larger schools and colleges of osteopathy run teaching clinics where you can have low-cost treatment from supervised students. These include: London College of Osteopathic Medicine (doctors only) Tel (071) 262 1125, British School of Osteopathy Tel (071) 930 9254, British College of Naturopathy and Osteopathy Tel (071) 435 7830. European School of Osteopathy Tel (0622) 671 558.

POLARITY THERAPY

Practitioners train for two to three years part-time and use the initials MEA (Member of the Energetics Association), MISPT (Member of the International School of Polarity Therapy) and RPT (Registered Polarity Therapist) according to which college they attended. For a list of practitioners, send £1 to the British Polarity Council, Monomark House, 27 Old Gloucester Street, London WC1N 3XX.

PSYCHOTHERAPY

Counselling and psychotherapy are sometimes available on the NHS, so ask your GP about local practitioners. Otherwise, there are approximately 1000 centres in the UK offering private counselling. Some are specialised, such as the Institute of Family Therapy and branches of Relate for marriage and partnership guidance, but others, like the Westminster Pastoral Foundation and the Tavistock Clinic, both in London, offer a wide range of support, some of it on the NHS. *Be warned*, however: charitable and Government-subsidised institutions are usually over-subscribed and waiting lists are long.

At present, anybody can attend a weekend course and call themselves a 'psychotherapist' or 'counsellor'. The National Register of Psychotherapists of the United Kingdom Council for Psychotherapy (UKCP) lists accredited practitioners working to a professional code of practice and ethics and subject to a complaints procedure. Training organisations must comply to certain standards. For further information contact the UKCP, Regent's College, Inner Circle, Regent's Park, London NW1 4NS. Tel (071) 487 7554.

The British Association of Psychotherapists (a member of the UKCP and the British Confederation of Psychotherapists) offers an assessment consultation for a fee of £35, and will try to find a suitable practitioner among its members. Sessions with a psychoanalytical psychotherapist are upwards of £20 for 50 minutes, depending on where you live. There is a reduced fee scheme, on a sliding scale of £6 to £13 per session. Contact the British Association of Psychotherapists, 37 Mapesbury Road, London NW2 4HJ. Tel (081) 452 9823.

The British Association of Counselling, which has close links with the UKCP, publishes a resource directory listing counselling and psychotherapy centres as well as individual practitioners in private practice, according to region. All members must comply with the Association's code of ethics.

Send a large stamped addressed envelope to the British Association for Counselling, 1 Regent Place, Rugby, Warwickshire CV21 2PJ. Tel (0788) 578 328.

Other useful addresses: Westminster Pastoral Foundation,
23 Kensington Square, London W8 5HN. Tel (071) 937 6956.
Tavistock Clinic, 120 Belsize Lane, London NW3 5BA.
Tel (071) 435 7111. Relate, Herbert Gray College, Little Church
Street, Rugby CV21 3AP. Tel (0788) 573 241. See telephone
directory for local centres.

QI GONG

There is no overall qi gong organisation in the UK at present. For
further information contact the Healing Tao Foundation (England),
P.O. Box 195, 85 Marylebone High Street, London W1M 3DE. Tel
(071) 224 1817 or the Community Health Foundation, 188-196 Old
Street, London EC1V 9FR. Tel (071) 251 4076.

RADIONICS AND RADIESTHESIA

Practitioners do four years of part-time training and use the letters
MRadA. Contact the Confederation of Radionics and Radiesthetic
Organisations, c/o The Maperton Trust, Wincanton, Somerset
BA9 8EH. Tel (0963) 32651.

REFLEXOLOGY

The newly-formed professional body, the Therapy Group for
Reflexology, is a member of the BCMA and adheres to its code of
practice. A register and minimum training standards are being
established. Although teaching is not extensive (60 hours is average),
subsequent experience is important, and many nurses are learning
reflexology.

For details of qualified practitioners, contact The British Reflexology
Association, Monks Orchard, Whitbourne, Worcester WR6 5RB.
Tel (0886) 821207.

The Association's official teaching body is the Bayly School of
Reflexology, whose graduates can apply for membership after a
year in practice, which authorizes them to use the title Registered
Reflexologist and the letters MBRA. Members have insurance cover.

Send £1.50 for a register of UK members. Association of Reflexologists, 25 Friars Walk, Lewes BN7 2LF. Tel (0273) 479 020.

The AR is open to reflexologists from one of their accredited schools, who agree to follow the Association's rules and ethical code. Minimum training is nine months, part-time, with 60 hours experience. Full members use the letters MAR.

RELAXATION AND BREATHING

A number of complementary therapies – massage, aromatherapy, shiatsu – induce a state of relaxation, but learn to slide into it yourself. Attend a class if there is one locally, but there are also a number of tapes available that talk you through a relaxation session, such as the British Holistic Medical Association's Tapes for Health, available from British Holistic Medical Association, 179 Gloucester Place, London NW1 6DX. Tel (071) 262 5299.

ROLFING

Because of the intimacy of the positions you find yourself in, it is important that there is a trusting relationship between yourself and the practitioner. Rolfers train over an 18-month period through the Rolf Institute, whose headquarters are in Boulder, Colorado, USA. For further information about Certified Rolfers contact Jennie Crewdson on (071) 834 1493.

SHIATSU

The Shiatsu Society keeps a register of members who have completed a recongised course of training (minimum length three years) and have satisfied the Society's assessment panel. Contact the Shiatsu Society, 5 Foxcote, Wokingham, Berks RG11 3PG. Tel (0734) 730 836.

SOUND THERAPY

Although sound is acknowledged to be implicated in health, there are few practitioners working in this field. For further information about cymatics contact Dr Peter Manners, Bretforton Hall, Bretforton, Vale of Evesham, Worcs WR1 5JH. Tel (0386) 830 537. Practitioners charge £30 for an initial interview, diagnosis and treatment, and thereafter £20 an hour.

T'AI CHI CH'UAN

Some information about classes and teachers may be available from the School of T'ai chi Ch'uan, 5 Tavistock Place, London WC1H 9SN. Tel (081) 444 6445. Local libraries, health clubs, community centres and newspapers sometimes advertise T'ai chi classes, but check the teacher's experience.

THERAPEUTIC TOUCH

It is not easy to find a TT practitioner within the NHS, as few nurses will openly offer to practise it. It is always worth asking though; you could be pleasantly surprised.

Otherwise, contact the Didsbury Trust, Sherborne Cottage, Litton, near Bath, Avon BA3 4PS. Tel (0761) 241 640.

TRADITIONAL CHINESE MEDICINE

Finding a qualified practitioner is vital, especially if you are prescribed acupuncture or herbal medicine. Just because a practitioner claims to have trained in China is not proof of competence. Qualified practitioners are registered members of the Council for Acupuncture, which represents five bodies who have agreed training standards and codes of ethics and practice (see *Acupuncture*) and publishes a directory of accredited British acupunturists. To receive this, send a stamped addressed envelope and £3 to the Council for Acupuncture, 179 Gloucester Place, London NW1 6DX. Tel (071) 724 5756 Fax (071) 724 5330.

To find a qualified herbalist with two years minimum training, contact the Register of Chinese Herbal Medicine, 21 Warbeck Road, London W12 8NS.

VISUALISATION

In everyday situations where you might need an extra boost of self-confidence or motivation, most of us can try visualisation for ourselves. Some claim success in mentally shrivelling warts. However, in cases of disease or psychological conditions, it is advisable to get professional help. There are no visualisation practitioners as such, but many behavioural psychotherapists and counsellors employ the technique as part of their treatment (see *Psychotherapy and Counselling*).

VOICE THERAPY

Paul Newham founded Voice Movement Therapy, and trains many of the therapists in the UK. For further information or a list of therapists, send a stamped addressed envelope to the International Association for Voice Movement Therapy, 7c Ballards Lane, Finchley, London N3 1UX. Tel (081) 693 9202.

Jill Purce, a musical healer, leads workshops in ancient vocal techniques and the spiritual potential of voice in healing and meditation. For further information, contact Inner Sound, 8 Elms Avenue, London N10 2JP. Tel (081) 444 4855.

YOGA

Western teachers are bringing fresh insights to the techniques. Training courses vary, from one to two years part-time. For further information about classes, contact the British Wheel of Yoga, 1 Hamilton Place, Boston Road, Sleaford, Lincolnshire NG34 7ES. Tel (0529) 306 851. Iyengar Yoga Institute, 223a Randolph Avenue, London W9 1NL. Tel (071) 624 3080. Yoga For Health Foundation, Ickwell Bury, Biggleswade, Bedfordshire SG18 9EF. Tel (0767) 627 271.

The Yoga Therapy Centre at the Royal London Homeopathic Hospital, 56-57 Great Ormond Street, London WC1N 3HR. Tel. (071) 833 7267 runs clinics for those suffering from asthma, diabetes and hypertension as well as back pain and can provide details of trained yoga therapists in other parts of the UK.

For general advice or information about complementary medicine or the registering bodies, there are a number of organisations who may be able to help. These include:

British Holistic Medical Association (BHMA), 179 Gloucester Place, London NW1 6DX. Tel (071) 262 5299 (doctors, health professionals and members of the public working for a change in attitude and the way healthcare is delivered through the NHS and private practice). Natural Medicines Society (NMS), Edith Lewis House, Ilkeston, Derbyshire DE7 8EJ (protects the present existence and future development of natural medicines). Research Council for Complementary Medicine (RCCM), 60 Great Ormond Street, London WC1N 3JF. Tel (071) 833 8897 Fax (071) 278 7412.

There are also a number of so called umbrella bodies which purport to represent some sections within complementary medicine. Not all the groups or disciplines subscribe to umbrella groups, with many of the more established professions preferring to operate their own registration and representative schemes. The experience of the Department of Health with umbrella groups has resulted in it preferring to have contacts with each profession on an individual and group-by-group basis. The umbrella organisations are:

British Complementary Medicine Association (BCMA), St Charles Hospital, Exmoor Street, London W10 6DZ. Tel (081) 964 1205 Fax (081) 964 1207. Council for Complementary and Alternative Medicine (CCAM), 179 Gloucester Place, London NW1 6DX. Tel (071) 724 9103. Institute for Complementary Medicine (ICM), PO Box 194, London SE16 1QZ, Tel (071) 237 5165 Fax (071) 237 5175.

WHAT THE LETTERS STAND FOR

ACHO	Affiliation of Crystal Healing Organisations
AHO	Association of Hydrotherapy Organisations
AMA	Anthroposophical Medical Association
AOC	Aromatherapy Organisations Council
AR	Association of Reflexologists
AST	Association for Systematic Kinesiology
ATA	Association of Tisserand Aromatherapists
ATC	Aromatherapy Trade Council
BAc	Bachelor of Acupuncture
BAAB	British Acupuncture Accreditation Board
BAAR	British Acupuncture Association and Register
BAAT	British Association of Art Therapists
BAC	British Association for Counselling
BAP	British Association of Psychotherapists
BCA	British Chiropractic Association
BCMA	British Complementary Medicine Association
BCNO	British College of Naturopathy and Osteopathy
BCP	British Confederation of Psychotherapists
BHMA	British Holistic Medical Association
BMAS	British Medical Acupuncture Society
BNOA	British Naturopathic and Osteopathic Association
BPSS	British Society of Psychotherapists
BRA	British Reflexology Association
BRI	British Register of Iridologists
BSD	British Society of Dowsers
BSECH	British Society of Experimental and Clinical Hypnosis
BSMDH	British Society of Medical and Dental Hypnosis
BSO	British School of Osteopathy
BWOY	British Wheel of Yoga
CA	Council for Acupuncture
CCAM	Council for Complementary and Alternative Medicine
CHO	Confederation of Healing Organisations
CHP	Certificate in Hypnotherapy and Psychotherapy
CO	College of Osteopaths
COA	Cranial Osteopathic Association
CPS	College of Psychic Studies
CRAH	Central Register of Advanced Hypnotherapists

CSAS	Chung San Acupuncture Society
DC	Diploma in Chiropractic
DHom	Diploma in Homeopathy
DipAc	Diploma in Acupuncture
Dip Phyt	Diploma in Phytotherapy (Herbal Medicine)
Dip THP	Diploma in Therapeutic Hypnosis and Psychotherapy
DO	Diploma in Osteopathy
DrAc	Doctor of Acupuncture
DSH	Diploma from the School of Homeopathy
DTM	Diploma in Therapeutic Massage
EA	Energetics Association
ESO	European School of Osteopathy
FBAcA	Fellow of the British Acupuncture Association
FBRA	Fellow of the British Reflexology Association
FFHom	Fellow of the Faculty of Homeopathy
FNIMH	Fellow of the National Institute of Medical Herbalists
FRH	Fellow of the Register of Herbalists
FTA	Floatation Tank Association
GCRN	General Council and Register of Naturopaths
GCRO	General Council and Register of Osteopaths
GOsC	General Osteopathic Council
IACT	International Association of Colour Therapy
ICM	Institute for Complementary Medicine
IFA	International Federation of Aromatherapists
IMH	Institute of Medical Herbalists
ISPA	International Society of Professional Aromatherapists
ITEC	International Therapy Examination Council
KF	Kinesiology Federation
LCH	Licentiate of the College of Homeopathy
LicAc	Licentiate in Acupuncture
LNCP	Licentiate in the National Council of Psychotherapists and Hypnotherapy Register
MAc	Master of Acupuncture
MAR	Member of the Association of Reflexologists
MBAcA	Member of the British Acupuncture Association
MBCA	Member of the British Chiropractic Association
MBEOA	Member of the British European Osteopathic Association
MBNOA	Member of the British Naturopathic and Osteopathic Association

MBRA	Member of the British Reflexology Association
MBRI	Member of the British Register of Iridologists
MBSA	Member of the British School of Acupuncture
MBSR	Member of the British School of Reflexology
MCA	McTimoney Chiropractic Association
MCH	Member of the College of Homeopathy
MCO	Member of the College of Osteopaths
MCOA	Member of the Cranial Osteopaths Association
MCROA	Member of the Cranial Osteopathic Association
MEA	Member of the Energetics Association
MFG	Member of the Feldenkrais Guild
MFHom	Member of the Faculty of Homeopathy
MH	Master Herbalist
MIACT	Member of the International Association of Colour Therapists
MIFA	Member of the International Federation of Aromatherapists
MIPC	Member of the Institute of Pure Chiropractic
MIROM	Member of the International Register of Oriental Medicine
MISPT	Member of the International Society of Polarity Therapists
MNAHP	Member of the International Association of Hypnotists and psychotherapists
MNCP	Member of the National Council of Psychotherapists and Hypnotherapy
MNIMH	Member of the National Institute of Medical Herbalists
MRadA	Member of the Radionics Association
MRCHM	Member of the Register of Chinese Herbal Medicine
MRH	Member of the Register of Herbalists
MRN	Member of the Register of Naturopaths
MRO	Member of the Register of Osteopaths
MRSS	Member of the Register of the Shiatsu Society
MRTCM	Member of the Register of Traditional Chinese Medicine
MSS	Member of the Shiatsu Society
MSTAT	Member of the Society of Teachers of the Alexander Technique
MTAS	Member of the Traditional Acupuncture Society
NCRI	National Council and Register of Iridologists
ND	Diploma in Naturopathy
NFSH	National Federation of Spiritual Healers
NIMH	National Institute of Medical Herbalists

NMS	Natural Medicines Society
NRHP	National Register of Hypnotherapists and Psychotherapists
RAH	Register of Advanced Hypnotherapists
RATh	Registered Art Therapist
RCCM	Research Council for Complementary Medicine
RIR	Registered Iridologist
RMTh	Registered Music Therapist
RPT	Registered Polarity Therapist
RSHom	Registered with the Society of Homeopaths
RTCM	Register of Traditional Chinese Medicine
SRMTh	State Registered Music Therapist
STAT	Society of Teachers of the Alexander Technique
UKCP	United Kingdom Council for Psychotherapy

GLOSSARY OF TERMS

AURA

An energy field that is said to radiate from all living organisms – humans, animals, plants and even crystals. Some people claim to be able to see auras, and to diagnose the physical, emotional and spiritual condition of an individual by the colour, shape and intensity of their aura.

BODYWORK

A general term for therapies that work with the body. These come under four headings:

energetic techniques activate the body's vital force or self-healing powers, as in acupuncture and yoga.

mechanical techniques include all kinds of massage and manipulation.

psychological techniques exercise the body to affect the mind, and the mind to affect the body, as in bioenergetics.

integrative techniques explore and enhance the interaction between mind, body and spirit, as in t'ai chi ch'uan.

CANDIDA ALBICANS

A fungus that favours warm, moist places and normally lives in the gut and often the mouth and vagina. Occasionally it runs amok and causes disease. This can manifest as a local infection, known as thrush, or less obviously as general ill health or allergies. People whose *immune systems* are suppressed are particularly vulnerable, such as babies, the elderly, diabetics, those taking antibiotics or steroids, and those suffering from AIDS.

CHAKRAS

In Sanskrit, the ancient Hindu language, *chakra* means 'wheel'. According to Hindu mystics, there are seven chakras – spinning centres or vortices – along the spinal column through which universal life energy (*prana*) interacts with the body and mind. To maintain physical, emotional and spiritual health, these centres should spin evenly and in harmony.

Each chakra is associated with certain emotions, colours, aromatic oils and gemstones which are said to help restore balance when the chakra is disrupted. The crown chakra (purple) on the top of the head is associated with bliss and spirituality; the brow chakra (indigo), the 'third eye' above the nose, with intuition and imagination; the throat chakra (blue) with creativity and assertiveness; the heart chakra (green) with love; the solar plexus chakra (yellow) with power; the sacral chakra (orange), just above the pubic bone, with sexuality; and the root chakra (red), behind the genitals, with fear and survival.

CHANNELLING

This refers to the process whereby individuals allegedly act as a channel or route for the expression of an external energy. Healers, for example, may believe they 'channel' power from a supreme source they could call God. Others might claim to 'channel' the spirit of a dead person, or of an extraterrestial being.

COMPRESS

A towel soaked in hot or cold water, wrung out and applied to the part of the body requiring treatment. A hot compress will increase blood flow and encourage sweating to flush out any toxins; a cold compress constricts blood vessels, restricting circulation and reducing inflammation.

ELIMINATION DIET

A method of testing for food allergies. Various foods are taken out of the diet to see what happens. If the allergic reaction stops, then the foods are re-introduced, one by one until the culprit is identified. The most common problem foods are milk and dairy products, wheat, coffee, chocolate, eggs and citrus fruits.

ENDORPHINS

Known as the body's natural painkillers, these opiate-like hormones are *neurotransmitters* (chemical messengers) that are found in the brain and spinal cord. An increase in endorphin levels can relieve pain and heighten feelings of pleasure. Recently, endorphins have been found in other parts of the body, including the immune system, encouraging the hypothesis that mind and body are more closely linked than realised.

ENKEPHALINS

Peptides (amino acid compounds) that have a painkilling effect similar to endorphins. Produced by nerve endings in the brain, these *neurotransmitters* are believed to have a sedative and mood-changing effect.

FIGHT OR FLIGHT

This is the initial response we make when confronted with a stressful situation. Our body goes into a state of arousal that will enable us either to tackle the aggressor or run away from it. Extra reserves of stress hormones – adrenalin, noradrenalin and cortisol – rush to all parts; blood pressure rises, the heart pumps faster; muscles tense; the liver releases sugar and fats for fast energy; the rate of breathing increases to provide more oxygen to power body tissues; blood clots more quickly, ready to seal injuries; digestion stops to divert all available energy to the muscles; saliva dries up; arteries constrict so that less blood is lost if wounded; perspiration increases. When you consider that all this can happen because of a traffic jam, the toll on the body leading to stress-related disease is not surprising.

IMMUNE SYSTEM

The body's defence against foreign substances (allergens); invading organisms such as bacteria, fungi and viruses; and its own abnormal cells, as in cancer and autoimmune diseases such as rheumatoid arthritis. The lymph nodes, spleen and thymus gland produce 'warrior' proteins known as antibodies, which can render these marauders harmless. They are helped by T cells, from the thymus, and by K or killer cells, which can directly destroy enemy cells (antigens). The different parts of the immune system 'talk' to each other through chemical messengers known as *neurotransmitters*.

KIRLIAN PHOTOGRAPHY

A technique that creates an electrical field so intense that electrons break away from surfaces. These can be recorded on a photographic plate and look like a halo or *aura* around an object. In dead objects, this halo is constant. Living objects (especially humans) show sudden flares and pulsations that are said to reflect the psycho-logical and physical state of the subject. The phenomenon was discovered by a Russian engineer, Semeyon Kirlian, and his wife, Valentina in 1939, but did not reach the West until the 1960s.

Innumerable claims have been made for the technique's potential as a diagnostic and counselling tool, but studies of sufficient rigour to satisfy scientists have only just begun.

LACTOBACILLUS ACIDOPHILUS
A friendly bacterium introduced into the gut to balance harmful bacteria, yeasts and fungi such as *Candida*.

MANDALA
An intricate pattern or design of Eastern origin, usually circular, that is used as an aid to meditation. In Buddhist and Hindu art, it often represented the universe; psychoanalyst, Carl Jung, saw it as a symbol of the integrated psyche.

MANIPULATION
Techniques practised by chiropractors, osteopaths, and physiotherapists which involve handling the patient's body to allow bone joints and soft tissues to move more freely, ease muscle spasm and relieve pain.

MANTRA
From the Sanskrit *man/tra*, 'instrument of thought'. Originally, a sacred word or group of words from the ancient Hindu writings, the Vedas, used in prayers and incantations. Now, a word or phrase repeated as an aid to meditation, so that extraneous thoughts are pushed out and the mind is able to focus. Some meditation schools claim that you must be 'given' a personal mantra, but most practitioners say that any word or words, even nonsense ones, will do.

MERIDIANS
In traditional Chinese medicine, these are invisible channels or pathways through the body along which Qi flows. There are said to be 14 main meridian channels that run to and from the hands and feet to the body and head, and along these are dotted acupuncture points where Qi is concentrated.

MOXIBUSTION
A technique for applying heat to acupuncture points to affect the flow of Qi. Moxa is the Oriental name for the plant, *Artemisia vulgaris*, a member of the chrysanthemum family. The dried leaves can be rolled into moxa sticks, and the moxa 'punk', a cotton-wool-

like fibrous substance, shaped into cones, both of which are burned directly over the points or on acupuncture needles. In a modern variation, the heat source can be electrical.

NEUROPEPTIDES
A group of *neurotransmitters* thought to be triggered by feelings.

NEUROTRANSMITTERS
Chemical messengers from the nerve endings that lock on to target cells throughout the body.

PLACEBO EFFECT
(From the Latin, 'I will please'). When any form of therapy or medicine is offered, 30 per cent of patients will report an improvement, even when there is no active agent involved in the treatment. Believing that something does you good seems to reap its own benefit. The effect often wears off with time, but in research studies it must always be accounted for. It is extraordinarily powerful: in a study of anti-ulcer drugs, 50 to 60 per cent of ulcers healed with a placebo during a six week period, compared with about 70 per cent using the real drug. Some researchers argue that this power of the mind over physical and psychological health should be taken more seriously.

PRANA
Universal energy associated with the breath that is believed to be absorbed into the body through the *chakras*, and maintains well-being. The concept is very similar to that of Qi.

PSYCHONEUROIMMUNOLOGY (PNI)
Leading-edge study of the mind–body connection, and the links between psychology, neurophysiology, and immunology. It is possible that our feelings may affect the action of *neurotransmitters* and the messages they carry to the *immune system* and the nervous system. This would mean that our emotions could have an impact on our health, and vice versa.

QI
Pronounced chee, in traditional Chinese medicine this is the vital essence, the life energy that nourishes and protects the body. Our Qi is said to come from various sources – the air, the food we eat, and, prenatally, from our parents.

FURTHER READING

General

British Medical Association. *Complementary medicine – new approaches to good practice*, Oxford University Press (1993)

Fulder, S. *The handbook of complementary medicine*, Coronet (1988)

Gravett, P. *Making sense of English in alternative medicine*, W. & R. Chambers (1993)

Inglis, B. and West, R. *The alternative health guide*, Michael Joseph (1984)

Moyers, B. *Healing and the mind*, Thorsons (1993)

Reader's Digest, *Family guide to alternative medicine* (1991)

Sharma, U. *Complementary medicine today – practitioners and patients*, Tavistock/Routledge (1991)

Smyth, A. *Gentle medicine*, Thorsons (1994)

Specific subjects

Hall, N. M. *Reflexology – a way to better health*, Gateway Books (1991)

Hewitt, J. *The complete relaxation book*, Rider (1989)

Hodgkinson, L. *Spiritual healing*, Piatkus Books (1992)

Kaptchuk, T.J. *Chinese medicine*, Rider (1987)

Kenyon, Dr J, *Acupressure techniques*, Thorsons (1987)

LeShan, L. *How to meditate*, Thorsons (1993)

Lidell, L. *The book of massage*, Ebury Press (1993)

Lockie, Dr A. *The family guide to homeopathy*, Hamish Hamilton (1990)

Lockie, Dr A. and Geddes, Dr N. *The women's guide to homeopathy*, Hamish Hamilton (1993)

Mabe, R. and McIntyre, M. *The complete new herbal*, Elm Tree Books (1991)

Maxwell-Hudson, C. *The complete massage book*, Dorling Kindersley (1988)

McIntyre, A. *Herbal medicine*, Optima (1987)

McIntyre, A. *Herbs for common ailments*, Gaia Books (1992)

Ridolfi, R. *Shiatsu*, Optima (1992)

Ryman, D. *The aromatherapy handbook*, C.W. Daniel (1989)

Sandler, S. *Osteopathy*, Optima (1992)

Sutcliffe, J. *Relaxation techniques*, Headline (1993)

Tisserand, R. *Aromatherapy for everyone*, Penguin Books (1990)

Other books published by the Health Education Authority, available through all good bookshops or, in case of difficulty, through Marston Book Services (HEA orders), PO Box 87, Oxford OX2 0DT:

The Good Health Guide Dr Alan Maryon Davis

This is the ultimate guide to healthy living in the 1990s. It offers comprehensive information on all aspects of health with realistic advice on how to achieve a healthy lifestyle.

£6.99   ISBN 1 85448 987 9

Women's Health Guide Mary Tidyman and Anne Furedi

Whether you're 16 or 60, this book will give you valuable help and insight into how you can take control of your health. Covering every stage in a woman's life from menstruation to the menopause, it will help you to help yourself to better health.

£10.99   ISBN 1 85448 992 5

Men's Health Guide Dr Ian Banks

This is an essential medical guide written specifically for men. It offers comprehensive and up-to-date advice on all aspects of a healthy, balanced lifestyle.

£8.99   ISBN 0 7521 0165 X   Available October 1994